IMMUNIZATIONS:
THE PEOPLE SPEAK!

**Questions, Comments, and Concerns
About Vaccinations**

IMMUNIZATIONS:
THE PEOPLE SPEAK!

Questions, Comments, and Concerns About Vaccinations

By Neil Z. Miller

New Atlantean Press
Santa Fe, New Mexico

IMMUNIZATIONS: THE PEOPLE SPEAK!

Questions, Comments, and Concerns About Vaccinations

By Neil Z. Miller

International Standard Book Number:
1-881217-16-7
Library of Congress Catalog Card Number:
95-72728

Cataloging-in-Publication Data
Miller, Neil Z.
   Immunizations : the people speak! questions, comments, and concerns about vaccinations / by Neil Z. Miller.
   p. cm.
   Includes bibliographical references and index.
   ISBN 1-881217-16-7   95-72728

   1. Vaccination of children--Complications. 2. Immunization--Complications. 3. Communicable diseases in children. I. Title

RJ240.M55 1996   614.4'7

$8.95 Softcover

Printed in the United States of America

Published by:
New Atlantean Press
PO Box 9638
Santa Fe, NM 87504

TABLE OF CONTENTS

*This book is dedicated
to parents and children
everywhere.*

FOREWORD

By Dr. Robert C. Martin

Taking things for granted is a modern-day necessity. We have so much to consciously consider on a daily basis that we generalize as many conclusions as possible, pigeon-holing them out of the way. For some, we rely on observation and logic. If the car posed no problems on the way home, we expect it to get us to work the next day. For others, we turn to wishful thinking. We expect to enjoy ongoing good health, for example, while abusing our bodies.

Regardless of how we arrive at our conclusions, we are jolted into disbelief when events prove us wrong. The mind really does not want to admit that vital information may have been overlooked or ignored. This habit of mind may explain some of the discomfort you are likely to experience while reading this book.

For most Americans, vaccination is a closed subject — something else to take for granted. Vaccines are so widely accepted that public safety threats and alternative approaches are hardly ever considered newsworthy. Even the known risks of inoculation are accepted. Misled by the promise of continued good health in lieu of some dreaded disease, we have concluded we have no choice but to vaccinate our children. The possibility that other associated risks may exist rarely enters our decision-making process.

I consider myself forever indebted to professors Maxine McMullen RN, DC, and Virgil Strang DC, for alerting me to the risk factors of vaccines as well as opening my eyes to the existence of alternatives. Since 1972, my first year as a chiropractic student, my wife and I have had the privilege of raising six children. I regard their excellent health as vindication of my decision to defy the powers-that-be and raise them without inoculations.

Neil Miller has provided a valuable public service by going beyond mere statistics. He has "humanized" the numbers by sharing the voices of concerned parents, many of whom have witnessed the downside of inoculation. The Q&A format is straightforward, allowing you to consider the relevant risk factors and arrive at your own conclusions. You may be surprised by this information. You may wonder why it was not available before now. But I doubt you will ever again take the subject of vaccination for granted.

>Dr. Robert C. Martin
>Chiropractic Physician and
>Nationally Syndicated Host of "Health Talk"
>September 1995

P REFACE

By Neil Z. Miller

I have been researching vaccinations for several years now. My first two books, *Vaccines: Are They Really Safe and Effective? A Parent's Guide to Childhood Shots*, and *Immunization Theory vs. Reality: Exposé on Vaccinations*, contain documented studies and other significant data showing how vaccines may be unsafe and ineffective. Information in those books was gleaned mainly from medical resources, including well-respected scientific journals.

In this book, *Immunizations: The People Speak!*, my intent is to provide the reader with an honest cross-section of vaccination concerns. The questions, comments, and personal stories are real. Together, they paint a picture of the national mood regarding this enigmatic and controversial topic. My own feeling is that the American people are perplexed, desperate for honest information on which to base their decisions.

But honest data is hard to come by. While much of it is buried in the medical literature, some of it is deliberately suppressed from the American people — like the fact that the government operates a vaccine insurance fund to compensate parents when their children are damaged or killed by mandated vaccines. Is it any wonder we find it difficult to determine who or what to believe?

Recently, a pregnant mother shared with me the following story. She said that a close friend took her child to the clinic for her shots. Soon thereafter the child became deathly ill. Both mothers "investigated" the problem and discovered several other mothers who had similar experiences at local clinics. They concluded that the clinics offered "generic" vaccines and that they needed to go to a doctor for the "good stuff." Evidently, the glorified vaccination concept is so deeply ingrained in the American psyche, that the damage being done to our own children is readily discounted.

My hope is that the many questions and comments voiced in this publication will provide you with an intimate glimpse — both pro and con — of the issues surrounding vaccinations. May God bless you for seeking the truth, for taking personal responsibility for your decisions, and for wanting only the very best that this world has to offer for your innocent and trusting children.

ACKNOWLEDGMENTS

I wish to express my encouragement and support toward the many parents and other concerned people seeking answers to their vaccination queries. I also want to applaud the wise individuals who had the courage and foresight to investigate this subject prior to exercising their options. I am confident that preventive healthcare measures will evolve. For all of our children, the American notion of freedom, and future generations, thank you.

WARNING!

The decision of whether or not to vaccinate is a personal one. The author is not a health practitioner and makes no claims in this regard. Nor does the author recommend for or against vaccines. All of the information in this book is taken from other sources and documented in the Notes section. If you have any questions, doubts, or concerns regarding any of the information in this book, go to the original source. Then research this topic even further so that you can make a wise and informed choice.

Neil Z. Miller
January 1996

T HE PEOPLE SPEAK!

Questions, Comments and Concerns About Vaccinations

The information in this book was taken directly from several national radio and television interviews granted by the author. The interviews were conducted in major cities throughout the country, including New York City, Sacramento, San Antonio, Nashville, Denver, Salt Lake City, and Phoenix. Typically, each interview lasted one hour, although some ran longer. Some hosts were sympathetic to my point of view; others were skeptical or adversarial. For ten or fifteen minutes we would banter back and forth exchanging information. Then the phone lines were opened for listeners to call in with their questions and comments.

The callers were usually moms and dads, although holistic health practitioners and medical doctors also responded. At first, I didn't anticipate the national yearning for dialogue on this topic. But the phone lines were jammed on every show with concerned parents and other individuals eager to discuss all aspects of this enigmatic and "forbidden" topic. These shows provided a fertile environment for an honest exchange of vaccine information.

INTRODUCTION

Question. How did you became interested in vaccines and what led you to publish a book?

Neil Miller: It all began when my first child was born. I wanted to look into the issue, but I found a dearth of unbiased information. Upon further research, I discovered a startling number of studies that opposed the traditional belief that vaccinations are safe and effective. The more data that I gathered, the more I realized how important it was to share this information with others. I organized the information into a cohesive format, and the book, *Vaccines: Are They Really Safe and Effective? A Parent's Guide to Childhood Shots* [see pages 79 and 80], evolved from this process.

Q. What kind of research did you do? Who did you talk to? How did you get the information for your book?

NM: I began my research by cutting out newspaper clippings and magazine articles on vaccines. Then I scoured through scientific and medical journals at college and medical libraries. I spoke with doctors, nurses, and concerned parents. Everyone had something to share. My information came from all of these sources.

Q. What are your qualifications?

NM: My main qualification is that I was concerned about the issue so I researched the topic. I have a college education, and I can think for myself. Also, I am a father.

Q. Have your qualifications been questioned by doctors?

NM: I believe that credentials are irrelevant to the issue because I have seen medical doctors who spoke out against vaccines maligned and suppressed by pro-vaccinators as quickly and effectively as the average layperson with less apparent training. Information that is fully disclosed can stand on its own. Nevertheless, doctors have been the least likely to confront me on this issue. However, a well known pediatrician debated me on national radio. In Utah, I debated against Dr. William Atkinson, a medical epidemiologist at the Centers for Disease Control. And I recently engaged in a spirited debate with another pediatrician on the Phil Donahue Show.

Q. Are you an authority?

NM: No. I see myself more as a provider of highly consequential information. By the same token, my research has convinced me that there are no vaccine authorities. The concept is an illusion, not unlike the vaccine ideology.

Q. I notice that your book contains a warning informing your readers that you are not a health practitioner and that you don't make recommendations for or against the vaccines. So you're not telling people what to do. You're just making this information available. Is that correct?

NM: Yes, that's exactly true. I sincerely believe the American people are capable of making rational decisions on their own, provided all pertinent information is disclosed. I am not interested in making decisions for other people. That is why every significant claim in my book is documented from other sources. I encourage parents to substantiate the information.

POLIO

Q. When was the polio vaccine introduced? Was polio on the rise or fall?

NM: The polio vaccines were introduced during the 1950s. The paralytic form of polio — most cases of polio are not paralytic — and the rate of death from polio were both declining on their own by the time the vaccine was introduced.[1]

Q. How is the polio vaccine made?

NM: The oral polio vaccine is made with a live virus, incubated in the organs of a dead monkey, then "stabilized" by adding antibiotics and other substances to the concoction.[2,4]

Q. Can my unvaccinated child catch polio from playing with recently vaccinated children?

NM: The polio germ can remain in the vaccinated child's intestinal system for up to two months.[5] It is possible — but not probable — for children and adults who come into contact with the vaccinated child during that period of time to contract the disease.[6]

Q. I saw a TV show that talked about polio. It said the vaccine that causes polio is the oral type, that the traditional kind, from a syringe, has never caused polio. It also showed a documented case where somebody got the polio disease from holding a baby that had just received the oral vaccine.

NM: The oral polio vaccine is the main vaccine that children receive. There are two polio vaccines, one with the live polio germ and one with the dead, or inactivated, polio germ. When babies are vaccinated with the live polio germ, the virus can remain in their system for up to eight weeks. When a parent or a grandparent changes the babies' diapers, for example, they can contract the disease. This is how many cases of polio occur.[7]

Q. Imagine how many people would have contracted polio if we didn't have the polio vaccine. What's the ratio here? How many people contracted polio from the vaccine versus how many people who were vaccinated?

NM: What would you consider an acceptable ratio? How many people can we sacrifice to the polio vaccine before we say it's unacceptable?

Q. How many cases of polio were caused by the polio vaccine?

NM: Since 1979, every single case of polio in the United States was caused by the polio vaccine.[8]

Q. If every known case of polio that we have in this country right now is as a result of the vaccine, isn't that a testament to what the vaccine has done?

NM: Whether the polio vaccine is fully or partly responsible for the decline in polio, that's one issue. The other more immediate issue now is, do we still need it? Is the polio vaccine necessary when it's now responsible for every case of polio in the United States?

Q. I remember when I was a child we watched a movie about polio and how there was a big epidemic during the 1950s. The only way that they got that under control was through vaccinations. Is that right, or is that propaganda?

NM: Throughout this century, the incidence and severity of polio periodically peaked and declined on its own. After the vaccine was introduced, researchers and health officials took full credit for polio's imminent cyclical decline. Also, when the vaccine was introduced, officials changed the criteria for defining polio. They made it more difficult to diagnose cases by requiring laboratory confirmation. And they began labeling more cases as aseptic meningitis, an affliction virtually indistinguishable from polio. These ploys dramatically skewed polio statistics.[9,10]

Q. I just read that archeologists have uncovered a 4,000-year-old mass grave containing one of the earliest recorded cases of polio. But the polio vaccine wasn't available 4,000 years ago. So if polio is that old and the vaccines weren't available, why doesn't everyone have polio? Why is it that polio wasn't more epidemic in our population?

NM: This seems to confirm what researchers have observed — that many of these diseases are cyclical in nature; they have their own natural rhythms. They enter a population and affect many people. Soon thereafter, large portions of the population gain a natural or "herd" immunity and become naturally immune. The disease then becomes relatively innocuous and may decline just as quickly, or "mysteriously," as it arose.[11]

Q. I have some information here saying that during the 1950s, even after the director of the New York Academy of Medicine announced that the immune serum against polio was known to

be dangerous and worthless, the National Institutes of Health continued to experiment with monkeys for three years using this identical serum. The serum was used, and several children died from it. However, the New York State Commissioner of Health at the time refused to hold hearings to investigate. There was a lot of political maneuvering to keep these things on the market.

NM: It is a well-known fact that the polio vaccine caused polio. Authorities knew this. There's been a remarkable cover-up and a lot of political maneuvering. In one study of the polio vaccine, when participants contracted the disease within 30 days of receiving the vaccine, no mention of this was made in the official records. Instead, those cases of polio were recorded as though they were contracted from the wild germ.[12,13] This kind of scheming and lying is well documented. A lot of these politics continue today.

Q. I remember as a young man in Southern California that we had very large polio wards. And I remember when the polio season came around how terrified everyone was that someone would get it. We don't have that anymore. The polio shots must be doing some good.

NM: Recently, several articles were published in well-respected journals, including *Lancet,* where researchers found that during the 1950s and 1960s more than 60 million people were inoculated with polio vaccines that were contaminated with monkey viruses. When they incubated the vaccines in monkey organs, undetected viruses were transferred to millions of people that received those polio vaccines. Today, scientists have found a link between at least one of these viruses and an increased incidence of cancer.[14-22] Evidence indicates we may be trading some diseases for others.[23-31]

Q. I was a polio pioneer. When I was a kid they lined up everybody from my school, and some kids got water and some kids got the actual Salk vaccine. I got the actual Salk vaccine. But I have friends who were born just three years before I was who didn't get the Salk vaccine. They're on crutches. I mean, polio's just something like, there it was, and there it wasn't.

NM: It's not that simple. Most of the people who contracted polio didn't get the paralytic form; of those that did, many were back on their feet within a brief period of time. More than 90 percent of the people who are exposed to the polio germ won't contract polio.[32] So there's some other factor operating there, perhaps nutrition.[33]

Q. I lived through that period when every neighborhood had two or three kids with polio. Our parents wouldn't even let us

go out to play with our friends. Swimming with other kids was unheard of. Your parents wouldn't let you do that. I also remember when they developed the vaccine, how happy everybody was, and the long lines at school where we got our vaccines. So I remember the dangers, and I remember how the vaccination program simply ended that almost overnight.

NM: I didn't live through that period, but I'm sure it was a scary time, perhaps like today with AIDS. But there are other factors involved. For example, the death rate from polio was decreasing on its own before the vaccine was discovered. In fact, from the early 1900s to the mid-1950s, the polio death rate in the United States and England decreased by more than 50 percent.[34] And when the polio vaccine was introduced, many European countries refused to systematically inoculate their citizens, yet polio epidemics ended in those countries as well.

Q. I'm old enough to remember when polio was a plague. As a kid, in every class that I had, there were several people that got polio, and it was feared. When Dr. Salk came out with his vaccine, the man was almost worshipped. People were dancing in the street. Before that time I used to see friends crippled with polio; some of them died. Since that time I've never seen a single case of it from my own experience. I'm willing to concede that there's risk in taking the shot, but isn't that risk much smaller than not taking the shot.

NM: That's the standard medical pitch. But there is another side to the issue. We need to look at vaccine safety, efficacy, and long-term effects, including what goes into the polio vaccine and how that's affecting the human constitution. Parents should be aware of all of the information that's out there, and they must remain free to choose whether or not they will vaccinate their children.

Q. I take issue when you say polio wasn't really that bad. If I understand you correctly, you're saying authorities manipulated statistics. I spent the last several years working with children from the Third World who do not get the vaccinations, and we have had many, many polio victims. It is *extremely* devastating. You can't tell me it doesn't exist and that you don't see that in other countries. So something must be helping.

NM: I don't mean to discount this terrible disease, or to deny that in Third World countries it may still be a problem. But many of these children are living in unsanitary environments. They are impoverished and malnourished. In 1949 there was an important study showing correlations between nutritional factors and polio.[35]

Other studies indicate that more than 90 percent of the people who are exposed to the natural polio germ will not contract the disease.[36] So we need to look at other factors, like the general health of the child and the sanitary conditions of the community. One of the problems, I think, is that medical intervention is promoted at the expense of these other important factors.

Q. You certainly wouldn't suggest Salk and Sabin were a bad thing?

NM: I believe that their brand of science — not polio — represents the greater scourge against society. Vaccine researchers at that time knew monkey viruses could contaminate vaccines, yet millions of children were inoculated with them.[37] And the polio vaccine caused polio in healthy kids.[38] This information was suppressed; it still is. Finally, I believe their dogma only served to inhibit research into genuine preventive measures, like the role of diet in disease.

MEASLES

Q. When I was growing up, we didn't have a measles vaccine. Everybody got the disease, and that was your way of being immune to it.

NM: I remember that too.

Q. What's wrong with getting measles? I had measles as a child, and I developed natural immunity.

NM: Exactly. It was no big deal. If the neighborhood children caught measles, our parents took us over so we would contract it as youngsters. Then we would be immune for life.

Q. It shocks me to hear doctors and health professionals talk about how dangerous measles and mumps were, and to talk about the death rates. I was shocked to hear about the number of people who died last year as a result of _measles_.

NM: Right.

Q. Measles and mumps were awfully benign diseases when I was growing up, even when my kids were growing up. We were expected to get the disease. Even our family doctor said, "Well, you know, he's got measles. Good. Keep him home for a week, and give him plenty of liquids and let it go at that." Nobody really thought much about it. Everybody got it. But in the last

ten years, I've started reading that physicians are now saying how dangerous these diseases are.

NM: At the turn of the century, measles was a critical disease. But by the time researchers developed the vaccine in the early 1960s, it was relatively benign. In fact, from 1915 to 1958, long before the first measles vaccine was introduced, a greater than 95 percent decline in the measles death rate had already occurred.[39] Some diseases, like measles, can be serious when they circulate through a virgin population — a group of people that hasn't been exposed to the germ. Complications and fatality rates are high. But once the population gains a herd immunity, it becomes a relatively tame illness.[40]

Q. Why?

NM: Because the population has been exposed to the wild germ and has gained a general immunity to it. But the measles vaccine started this cycle all over again by suppressing herd immunity. Now, when the wild measles germ shows up in the population, once again it's attacking virgin populations.[41]

Q. The sickest adult male I ever saw, who didn't die, was a man who had measles when he was about 26.

NM: Measles was a relatively innocuous disease by the time the vaccine was introduced. It occurred most often in toddlers. The vaccine changed that. Today, infants, teenagers, and adults are contracting the disease in record numbers — age groups more susceptible to extreme complications.[42]

Q. Is the measles vaccine effective?

NM: No. Today, when an outbreak of measles occurs you'll often hear scare tactics about how everyone needs to be vaccinated, as though low vaccination rates are causing the problem. But when you study the numbers, you'll find that up to 95 percent of the cases are in people who were vaccinated against measles.[43]

Q. My daughter is a freshman this year, and when I registered her for high school, they said that her MMR was out of date and she needed to have another one. But according to her records, she had two shots, one at the beginning of 1979 and one at the end of 1979.

NM: When the measles vaccine was first introduced, authorities touted it as a miracle cure. They claimed that one shot would protect for life, and that measles would be eradicated from the planet within a few years.[44] Obviously, vaccine policymakers will say anything to achieve their ends, and they rewrite the guidelines as they go along.

Q. At Fort Lewis College there was a measles outbreak. They immediately put all the students through a measles inoculation program. Lo and behold, two weeks later there was another outbreak, so they ran through the students again, but again two weeks later there was another outbreak. They quarantined all the kids in the elementary schools. Since my kids had not been vaccinated, they were sent home. Then Christmas break came, and even though the college was quarantined until Christmas break, all of a sudden kids were allowed to go home. A bunch of kids with fresh outbreaks of measles were allowed to return to all corners of the earth, yet my kids couldn't attend class.

NM: Your story is typical.

Q. I really think that we should take another look at vaccinating everyone. Fifteen years ago I was a mother who thought I had to do everything exactly right. So my kids were given all the shots. Well, there were two measles shots, a dead one and the live vaccine. One or the other, I forget now which it was, but they decided it wouldn't work. So both of my sons had to be revaccinated. At seven years of age, my one son developed an asthmatic condition, or allergy, and the doctor put him on desensitizing shots. By the time he reached 18, he developed a strange form of lymphatic leukemia. When we first heard about it, we thought, oh no, he's a tonsil baby and a vaccination baby. The researchers were very alarmed that he had two measles shots, because they felt the measles virus was closely related to blood diseases. If I would have known this, I would have said, "We will take our chance on the first measles shot only." Well, I think it's very wrong to see them demand that every child is vaccinated.

NM: I sympathize and agree with you. I really don't think they understand what they're doing.

Q. I often wonder how my children would have grown if they were left alone. You know, being a good mother, and thinking doctors knew best, you went to your pediatrician and trusted that he knew what he was doing. But my children are now in their 30s, and they're having problems asthmatic-wise and bone-wise, and with other things that may have developed anyway. But the measles vaccine was so new at that time. I

suppose they didn't understand or didn't know. It really rang a bell with me when the oncologist asked me about the vaccines. When I told him about the two measles shots, he was furious.

NM: He sounds like a wise doctor.

Q. I am a pediatrician and just want to say that the likelihood of getting measles encephalitis is ten times greater with the disease than with the vaccine. It was significant that in a recent epidemic, 19 people died as a result of measles, and that was out of only 25,000 kids. If you factor that by what could happen if not enough people are vaccinated, I think the likelihood is that a significantly greater number of people would die.

NM: How many of those people who contracted the disease were previously vaccinated?

Q. [No answer.] Of all of the kids with measles that I took care of two years ago, two died. And that was preventable if those kids had been adequately immunized and the kids they had come in contact with had been adequately immunized.

NM: That doesn't make sense. If your vaccine is so effective, it wouldn't be necessary for the kids they come in contact with to be vaccinated as well.

Q. It's very important to have your child immunized early against measles and mumps.

NM: The number of vaccine failures is so great that it's a shame the medical establishment continues along this course. In fact, the Centers for Disease Control confessed long ago that vaccinated people are 14 times more likely to contract measles than people who are not vaccinated.[45]

Q. Is it ethical to allow young children to undergo the sickness and potential risk of dying from a disease that we have the ability to prevent them from getting?

NM: I'm not so sure that we have the ability to prevent them from getting the disease.

Q. Let's assume for just a second that we do. Even with a 50 percent efficacy, is it ethical to say, "We want you to go ahead and get the disease to gain a 'natural immunity?'" Is it ethical to allow somebody to get sick from something that we have a way to prevent?

NM: First of all, we have to seriously look at whether we truly do have a way to prevent the disease. Secondly, I would ask a similar question: Is it ethical to demand that people submit to certain health practices they may not agree with? Parents of vaccinated children often ask parents of unvaccinated children, "How will you feel if your child gets the disease?" This question can be reversed: "How will you feel if your child gets the vaccine and still comes down with the disease, or comes down with something worse as a result of the vaccine?"

Q. That really doesn't answer the question, though. Do you feel it's OK if your children come down with measles when you know there may be a way to prevent it?

NM: Yes. I think it's more important for them to derive natural immunity than taking a risk on the vaccine. In fact, several studies indicate that the immune system is strengthened by contracting diseases like measles. It may be nature's way of building resistance to fight off other diseases in the future.[46,47]

Q. Even though you yourself have recognized that measles may be a more dangerous disease today than it was 30 years ago?

NM: Yes. We also need to look at who is contracting measles. In many cases we're looking at children who are malnourished. Not enough emphasis is being placed on proper nutrition so that our children's immune systems will be strengthened to fight off disease when it enters the population.

RUBELLA

Q. What is rubella?

NM: Rubella, also known as German measles, is a relatively tame illness unless contracted by a pregnant woman.

Q. What happens when pregnant women contract rubella?

NM: When rubella is contracted by a pregnant woman during her first trimester, the child has a chance of being born with physical or mental defects.

Q. Is the rubella vaccine effective?

NM: Studies indicate the vaccine may only be effective for a few years.[48,49] So a girl who's been vaccinated against rubella at the age of four or five may no longer be protected by the time she reaches childbearing age.

Q. Is the vaccine safe?

NM: Recent independent studies show correlations between the rubella vaccine and chronic fatigue syndrome.[50] And women who receive the vaccine maintain an increased risk of contracting rheumatoid arthritis.[51]

Q. How soon after the child is vaccinated will chronic fatigue syndrome start to develop?

NM: It appears that adults who come in contact with the recently vaccinated child are the ones at risk. They are subjected to the virus emanating from the child. It enters the body and affects the immune system.[52]

Q. Are you saying that the child can precipitate somebody else's disease? Is that what you mean?

NM: Yes. The live rubella virus emanating from the child may be inhaled by adults they come in close contact with.[53] It's no different from polio where cases of the disease may occur in adults who come in close contact with a recently vaccinated baby.[54]

TETANUS

Q. The one shot that you always got questioned on, and you still do if you show up with even a scratch on your hand at any medical facility, is the tetanus shot. But some of the people who contract the disease have been adequately vaccinated. What does that tell us?

NM: It tells us that the vaccine may not be effective.

Q. What do you think about tetanus and the tetanus vaccine?

NM: I believe the dangers associated with contracting tetanus, and the efficacy of the tetanus vaccine, are exaggerated. During World War II, twelve cases of tetanus were recorded. Four of these cases — 33 percent — occurred in military members who were properly vaccinated.[55] No one really knows how well the tetanus vaccine helped to decrease the incidence of the disease because the tetanus vaccine was introduced at a time when we also began to have a greater understanding of wound hygiene.

Q. I remember seeing an old movie from the 1950s all about the first doctor who was adamant against operating with dirty hands. He insisted on creating a sterile environment. They laughed at him at the time and thought he was a kook.

NM: The tetanus spore requires precise conditions to grow and cause harm.[56] In my estimation wound hygiene is more significant than a vaccine.

PERTUSSIS

Q. Which vaccine is the worst?

NM: Many people believe the pertussis vaccine takes that dubious honor.

Q. The pertussis vaccine protects a kid against what?

NM: It was designed to protect against whooping cough, but its efficacy rate is poor. For example, in a recent epidemic, more than 70 percent of the cases were in children vaccinated against the disease.[57] And although whooping cough is generally not a serious disease unless it's contracted by infants,[58] the dangers of the pertussis vaccine have been known for decades, and are well documented in the scientific and medical literature throughout the world.[59]

Q. What is the acellular pertussis vaccine?

NM: It is a new vaccine for whooping cough that some researchers claim is less reactive than the current pertussis shot used in the United States. But some officials believe it is too expensive to replace our current, unpredictable vaccine.[60]

Q. I'm a pediatrician, and I warrant there are local side effects from the pertussis vaccine that are of some concern, meaning some irritation around the site of the shot, and in a very small fraction of doses, some indication and evidence that there may be a seizure associated with that. But all you have to do is look at situations where [vaccinations] have either lapsed or gotten to where the percentage of kids adequately [vaccinated] has fallen to such a low level, see the research of these, and you'll see the people who have been objecting to the vaccines come quickly trying to find vaccines for their child. The British have had that experience, the Japanese have had that experience, and the Swedes have had that experience. I would just as soon not see our country learn that lesson the hard way.

NM: When the British stopped vaccinating their children with the pertussis vaccine, cases of pertussis increased, but there were no increases in the death rate.[61] In fact, infant death rates plummeted.[62] When the Japanese stopped vaccinating their children with the pertussis vaccine, infectious disease rates dropped.[63] And the Swedes withdrew this vaccine from the market because of the dangers associated with it.[64]

Q. There was an extensive study that was released through the National Institutes of Health, and the FDA was a part of that study, which looked at the evidence that had been accumulated with respect to the DPT shot specifically, in terms of whether the side effects or the adverse outcome could be attributed to that particular vaccination. It was a review of the reviews. Clearly, the benefits outweigh the risks.

NM: Excuse me, but a "review of the reviews" is bogus when pertinent data is dismissed out of hand merely because it doesn't conform to expectations. Children die at a rate eight times greater than normal within three days after getting a pertussis vaccine.[65] Numerous studies have shown correlations between the pertussis vaccine and Sudden Infant Death Syndrome.[66,67] Additional evidence indicates the pertussis vaccine may be responsible for autism, hyperactivity, dyslexia, and other learning disorders.[68,69] And the *Journal of the American Medical Association (JAMA)* recently published a study showing that children with asthma were five times more likely than not to have been vaccinated with pertussis.[70] If what you say is true, then why did the government put together a program to compensate victims when they're damaged by the shots? And why has the government already paid millions of dollars to the parents of children damaged by this vaccine if it is so safe?[71]

Q. I happen to think the compensation program was an extremely humanitarian and appropriate thing to do for parents, so that the pharmaceutical companies wouldn't be sued, if there were in fact side effects or negative reactions.

NM: Your interest in the plight of the drug companies is laudable, but my point is that the government has already acknowledged, again and again, the dangers associated with this vaccine.

Q. I have four children. The oldest two never had a reaction to any of the vaccines. My third child, she's fair skinned and red haired, had what I consider to be a pretty severe reaction to her first two DPT shots. So of course we discontinued the vaccines. She's never had her MMR or the polio shots. Now it's time for my seven-month-old to get the shots. She was never vaccinated

because she has physical similarities to her sister — fair skin and red hair — and we were concerned. But my pediatrician has been urging me. He says that since the DPT caused the reaction, why don't I try the DT? Obviously, I'm scared.

NM: With good reason.

Q. I'm more concerned right now about the vaccines than the diseases themselves. I'm wondering, how valid is his point?

NM: You are a prime candidate for more information. You need to step out of the medical paradigm and read some of the unbiased vaccine information that is available. Then you will be able to make a wise decision for you and your family.

Q. I am a naturopathic physician, and I've run into this type of genetic makeup before. Fair-skinned, red-headed children often don't have the ability for their liver to break down the vaccine toxins. These are the same children who will not be able to handle drugs well, any drugs, including alcohol, and they have a tendency toward allergies. So there is a difference between the genetic makeup of these children and others in terms of how well their bodies are able to assimilate these toxins and break them down.

NM: Thanks for your input.

Q. I had whooping cough, and I would not recommend it to anybody. I was extremely ill, had a raging temperature, and two months after I was over the fever, I started to cough and vomit. I had absolutely no control. So I recommend getting the shot. I know people that said no, but my children were all vaccinated for it.

NM: Thanks for your input.

Q. I'm pretty sure that the pertussis vaccine caused seizures in two children that I'm very, very close to. Everything happened immediately after. The children were fine before. They were pulling up, talking, walking, doing everything a normal child would do.

NM: Until they received their pertussis shot?

Q. Yes. They got the DPT.

NM: And now the children are different?

Q. Yes. One is twenty with the mentality of an eight- or nine-year-old. The other boy can't walk or talk. He's about five. It breaks your heart. I just want to know, is there any way to prove this?

NM: The government has made it very difficult to prove these cases, and yet they are trying to mandate all vaccines. They refuse to spend time and money in trying to find out exactly how much damage is really being done out there.

Q. I'm a medical doctor, and I agree that it is an awful thing to have seizures happening in anybody. And if it was at all related to the immunizations, that also is terrible.

NM: Many of these cases are obviously related to the shots. But the medical establishment, and all its henchmen, live in denial.

Q. I am the manager of the State Immunization Program for the State Department of Health, and I just want to say that not only our state institution, but the Centers for Disease Control and Prevention, the American Academy of Pediatrics, and virtually every body of expert health professionals disagrees with virtually everything that you say. I think it's important for the public to know that.

NM: The public already knows that. That's why people like me are trying to make public the information that has been suppressed by people like you.

Q. Except that the studies you're referring to are not studies by reputable health professionals.

NM: Yes they are. Many come from the medical journals that you respect. But whenever a study comes out against vaccines, you and your cronies make every effort to discredit it by claiming, "This study is no good, because we refuse to validate it."

Q. Well, a previous caller was concerned about the risk associated with children not getting [vaccinated]. Let me just refer to the episode in Great Britain back between 1977 and 1979. During that two-year [three-year] period of time, there were approximately 100,000 cases of pertussis. That was because of concern about reactions associated with the vaccine.

NM: Let me explain, because you're not telling the whole truth. In 1975, in Great Britain, several people died from the pertussis vaccine. Parents stopped vaccinating their children, and two or three years later, cases of pertussis rose. But there were very few deaths. Although there were many cases of pertussis, very few children were dying. They were getting pertussis and passing through the disease.[72,73]

Q. Pertussis is a serious disease, whether or not a child dies. But let me also say that in the United States during that same period of time, we had 3,000 cases of pertussis [the true figure was 5,863][74] because our [vaccination] levels were around 90 percent, whereas in Great Britain they were 31 percent.

NM: And when vaccination rates dropped to 31 percent, infant mortality rates sharply declined![75]

SIDS

Q. What about SIDS — Sudden Infant Death Syndrome? What evidence have you collected on that illness?

NM: Studies throughout the world show correlations between the pertussis vaccine and critical adverse reactions, including Sudden Infant Death Syndrome.[76] Yet, whooping cough is rarely a serious disease unless contracted by infants.[77] In one study, performed by Dr. William Torch of the University of Nevada School of Medicine in Reno, out of 103 children who died of SIDS, 70 percent had received the DPT vaccine within three weeks.[78] Another study from Australia shows how young children experience stress-induced breathing patterns, including apnea — the cessation of breathing — immediately after receiving the pertussis vaccine, and these altered breathing patterns continue for up to two months following the shot.[79]

Q. You suggest there may be a link between some vaccines and Sudden Infant Death Syndrome. Is that true?

NM: Let me clarify; _I_ am not making these suggestions. Several studies by prominent researchers show what appear to be significant correlations between the pertussis vaccine and Sudden Infant Death Syndrome. Researchers throughout the world are concerned. And the U.S. government recently acknowledged that many of the cases in which parents were compensated for the deaths of their children due to vaccine-induced damage were originally classified as SIDS deaths.[80]

Q. When children have a fatal reaction to vaccines, they say the child died of SIDS. But SIDS is a syndrome, not a disease. It's a

conglomeration of things that happen to the body, caused by something. But they don't say what caused it, even if it only happened right after the child had the vaccine.

NM: That's true.

SMALLPOX

Q. I may be an uneducated layperson, but hasn't smallpox pretty much been eradicated from the earth?

NM: If you supplement your reading on smallpox with nonbiased information, you'll find that smallpox skyrocketed throughout the world only after smallpox vaccination campaigns were initiated. Conversely, smallpox deaths per capita tumbled only after the percentage of vaccinated babies dropped.[81]

Q. Smallpox is a disease that has been wiped out as result of vaccination. Right or wrong?

NM: Prior to 1796, the year Edward Jenner began experimenting with a smallpox vaccine, epidemics were small and limited. It was only after he came out with his vaccine that we began to have huge epidemics all over the world. The true figures indicate that an overwhelming number of people who contracted smallpox were actually vaccinated against the disease.[82]

Q. You talk about the number of people who got smallpox after they were vaccinated against the disease, but what about the millions of people who *didn't* get smallpox?

NM: Many wouldn't have gotten it whether they were vaccinated or not. And the medical establishment often changes the definition of a disease when a person contracts it after they were vaccinated. In other words, when people were vaccinated with the smallpox vaccine and came down with the disease, it was seldom listed as smallpox. They gave the disease a new name.[83] Again, smallpox epidemics ended only after people began refusing the shots.

HIB

Q. Our state and county health officials plan to inoculate 70,000 children against meningitis because 16 children caught the disease during the last few weeks, including a five-month-old

girl who died. The boundaries of the outbreak area were drawn up, and all children ages two to nine who are within the target area are eligible to receive free vaccines. Would you please comment on this?

NM: This is a common tactic used by the pediatric and medical associations. A few cases of a disease turn up and we have an "epidemic" on our hands. Then, everyone in the surrounding area must be vaccinated.

Q. So the meningitis vaccine is unnecessary?

NM: First of all, children can get meningitis from several types of germs. The Hib vaccine is designed to protect against meningitis arising from only one of these germs — haemophilus influenzae type B.[84] So, technically speaking, I wouldn't refer to it as the meningitis vaccine. Next, when a child contracts the Hib disease, it rarely causes full-blown meningitis. Instead, the child might experience upper respiratory distress, ear infections, or inflamed sinuses. The Hib shot is not designed to remedy any of these conditions.[85] Finally, you mention that children two to nine years old are eligible for the shot, but these children are *least* at risk for contracting the disease. Over 75 percent of all cases occur in children less than two years of age. The vaccine is not considered effective for children in this age group.[86,87]

Q. I have two kids, one 5 and one 9. My youngest had the Hib vaccination when she was in preschool; it was required. Now we're being told she needs to be vaccinated again. Is it the same vaccine, or is it something different?

NM: That's hard to say because during the last few years several different Hib vaccines were developed, licensed for use, tested on our children, and quietly withdrawn after it became clear they were either ineffective or dangerous. One in particular dramatically *increased* the odds of contracting the disease.[88]

Q. You mean it caused meningitis symptoms?

NM: Not the symptoms, but the actual full-blown disease. It was causing the exact conditions it was designed to prevent.

Q. So if she's already had this one, then it isn't going to be necessary for her to have it again? She's had it within the last two years.

NM: I don't make recommendations for or against the vaccines.

Q. Do you mean it's not going to do any more than it probably already did?

NM: That's an interesting way of putting it. I suppose it all depends on what you think it already did.

Q. My older daughter had a mild case of mononucleosis last year. I was told that when younger children have that, they are more susceptible to upper respiratory infections. She is almost 10 years old. Do you think she needs the Hib vaccine, or will her natural immune system take over for her?

NM: I don't make recommendations for or against vaccines, but I would suggest you remain cautious whenever scare tactics are employed. Look at the actual studies that were done on the efficacy and safety of the Hib vaccine.

Q. What really upsets me is the medical manipulation, whereby parents are frightened into allowing their children to be injected with substances they may be worried about, may not feel good about, or may know in their hearts are not going to be good for the child. That's where I have a problem.

NM: Recently, the American Academy of Pediatrics (AAP) tried to waive responsibility on this issue. Because of the controversy over the safety and efficacy of an earlier Hib vaccine — abandoned and replaced by "new and improved" versions — the AAP approved new guidelines recommending that doctors use their own discretion regarding whether or not to continue giving it to children.[89]

HEPATITIS

Q. I just finished a three-shot series of the hepatitis B vaccine. What is hepatitis, and what kind of dangers do I need to look out for with the vaccine?

NM: Hepatitis is a liver disease, usually accompanied by a fever, and linked to a virus. In one study, two-thirds of the doctors who were eligible for the hepatitis vaccine refused to take it.[90] That should be sufficient warning to the general population.

Q. After two of the shots, not all three of them, one of my co-workers got sick for a couple of days.

NM: Now authorities are trying to mandate this vaccine, and doctors are shooting up infants with it immediately after they're born, often without the parent's knowledge or consent.[91]

Q. Is it true that some babies are getting shots immediately after birth?

NM: Yes. Newborns are being injected with the hepatitis B vaccine — often without the parent's consent — in the hospital, right after birth.[92]

Q. Why?

NM: Medical policymakers haven't found a way to target high-risk groups — IV drug users. So doctors are injecting infants instead.[93]

PNEUMONIA

Q. I went for a physical in December, and they took my blood pressure and all of that. Then the doctor came up with the idea that I should have a pneumonia shot. I said, "I'd rather not take any shots at all." I had pneumonia in my 20s, but I never catch a cold or anything like that. Nevertheless, between his nurses and him, they finally got me to take the pneumonia shot. Well, two weeks later I got pneumonia. It was terrible. I was sick all during the Christmas holidays. I told my doctor, but he said no, that he didn't bring this on.

NM: I hear this all the time. You received the pneumonia vaccine, which is supposed to protect. Two weeks later you came down with pneumonia. And authorities deny that the vaccine caused it.

Q. They completely denied it. And not only that, the doctor charged Medicare $380 for that physical. If the government wants to take over our health plan, we'll really go bankrupt.

NM: I've read a study in which the pneumonia vaccine was shown to be ineffective.[94] In your case it apparently caused the disease.

Q. I'm 77 years old, and I have diabetes. I use insulin. About three weeks ago, I got pretty sick during the night and could hardly breathe. I went to the doctor the next morning and I had water on my lungs, with touches of pneumonia. I had it pretty well whipped, but it's starting to come back. Should I take the pneumonia shot?

NM: I am not a doctor. I am a research journalist and a natural health advocate. I don't make recommendations. However, you may be interested in a study that was published on the pneumonia vaccine. Of the 1,300 healthy children who participated in this study, half received the vaccine while the others were given a placebo. The authors of the study conclude there is no benefit from the pneumonia vaccine.[95]

Q. Why would doctors continue to recommend it?

NM: Doctors adhere to a certain belief system, a comfortable paradigm that they've established over time, and I believe they have a vested interest in maintaining that paradigm.

INFLUENZA

Q. Right now we're getting inundated in the news with why it's necessary for _everyone_ to go out and get a flu shot. Have you noticed that this year health officials say we're bracing for a particularly bad influenza season? It seems I heard this last year and the year before that. What do you think?

NM: I'm astonished that people continue to respond.

Q. A lot of people are just like sheep. They bow their heads and get the flu shot, never asking whether it's really necessary, if it has side effects, or if it is normal.

NM: It's a predictable response when people in power, like Donna Shalala, claim that up to 45,000 U.S. citizens per year die from the flu.[96] That is an extreme fabrication. It's just not true.

Q. I am a health practitioner. Right now there are a lot of folks coming into my office asking me for advice on the flu vaccine. I never tell them what to do. I just tell them to read and consider, and if in doubt, don't, when it comes to doing things they know little or nothing about and taking chances that may be unnecessary. Ultimately it's the individual's decision whether to get a flu shot or not. What's your opinion?

NM: I think it's interesting that every year authorities endorse a new flu vaccine designed to combat a new flu strain soon to arrive. This year it's the Beijing strain. I'd like to know how they know which strain will arrive, and how it's going to get here, especially when you consider that it normally takes several years, sometimes more than several decades, to develop a vaccine.

Q. We're talking about one vaccine for one strain of one virus.

How many viruses are estimated to be known today?

NM: Probably thousands.

Q. How do they know which one to make, then?

NM: Good question. This particular vaccine, by the way, is not only for the Beijing strain. The manufacturers must have had some leftover stock from previous years, because they also threw in the viruses for the Panama flu and for the Texas flu as well.[97]

Q. Do you know anything about the viruses they're using in the current flu vaccines?

NM: The new flu vaccine uses an "inactivated" virus — a "dead" virus. Dead virus sounds repugnant, so authorities say inactivated. The "inactivated" polio vaccine during the 1950s was allowed to contain a small percentage of the live polio germ, and was therefore capable of causing polio in people who received it.[98]

Q. It sounds to me like lite beer, or decaf.

NM: It's all a matter of propaganda and promotion.

Q. Authorities are saying that since the new flu vaccine is made with an inactivated, or dead, virus, people cannot get the flu as a result of taking it. Is this true?

NM: You should be aware of some of the tactics that are used to cover up side effects from the vaccine. For example, in yesterday's paper, an article on the flu vaccine mentioned that the inactivated virus cannot give you the flu. In the very next sentence the authors note that "some individuals might develop a mild fever and feeling of malaise for a day or two after the shot."[99] Correct me if I'm wrong, but isn't that the flu?

Q. It sounds just like the flu.

NM: Authorities are not coming right out and telling you that if you take their flu vaccine you may get the flu. If they were honest, everybody wouldn't be lining up like sheep.

Q. I think a lot of people believe there's a guarantee that they won't get the flu if they take the flu shot, and that's just not true. If you read it anywhere, I want to see it in print.

NM: It's absolute fraud trying to convince people they're not going to get sick from the so-called inactivated vaccine. It's all hype, its promotion. Authorities know that in the past people were afraid of the live virus, so they've come up with a new promotional tactic.

Q. What about the Swine flu?

NM: A few years ago more than 500 people who received a Swine flu shot were paralyzed with Guillain-Barré syndrome; more than 30 of them died.[100]

Q. I recently learned that in 1918, during the first World War, shots for influenza were compulsory for all servicemen. In that same year, the great flu epidemic occurred. Military hospitals were filled with many more casualties of the flu vaccine than of the war. Then authorities tried to mask the name. They called it the Spanish influenza. That was an attempt to conceal its origin.

NM: Tactics like this are not uncommon. Authorities did the same thing with polio when the polio vaccine was introduced; they diagnosed new polio cases as aseptic meningitis.[101]

Q. I've had so many respiratory problems in the last five weeks that I really wonder whether maybe this is the year I ought to take the flu shot. I'm literally afraid to take it but I got a call from a friend who said, "You know, thousands of people, tens of thousands of people, are going to die," and she was urging me. I really need to consider taking it. I had another friend call me to say, "You know, it's not a live virus — you're not going to get sick," and I'm thinking, well, should I take it, because a light case of the flu is better than a full-blown case. And I really need to consider it.

NM: You appear tormented, but you are the only one who can make that decision. I think that a lot of times it boils down to our belief systems. If you place your faith in the medical approach to health, that may very well be the best option for you. For others who are leery of the medical approach and who believe there are alternative ways to achieve natural immunity, that would be the way to go. You're just going to have to sit quietly with yourself to resolve this.

Q. Louisiana had three cases of the flu early in the season — three whole cases. I wonder if these are people who take care of themselves. Are these people who drink a lot of alcohol and lower their resistance? Is that why they came down with the flu? And is it in fact a flu to begin with, based on the fact that ailments are misdiagnosed about 60 percent of the time?

NM: It's hard to say, but I agree with your implication that a poor diet may contribute to the onset of disease.

Q. Have they changed anything about the flu shots? I had the flu about ten years ago after I got the flu shot.

NM: Every year authorities come out with a new flu shot because a new strain is expected to arrive. In one study of adults questioning whether to take the flu vaccine, over 50 percent of their doctors recommended against it.[102]

Q. For a ten-year period, every year I took the flu shot, along with a lot of other people at the company where I worked. For ten years we didn't get the flu. I hear these stories about people having adverse reactions, and I know they occur. But it just doesn't happen in my little territory.

NM: Again, that's why the entire issue boils down to freedom of choice. If you feel more comfortable getting the shots, you should be entitled to do that. And if others feel differently, they should be free to exercise their decisions as well.

LONG-TERM EFFECTS

Q. What are the long-term implications of injecting live viruses and foreign matter into the body?

NM: Concerned parents often consider the immediate consequences of vaccinating their children, but long-term studies on the vaccines are rarely conducted. Our children are medical guinea pigs because we just don't know the long-term ramifications of injecting a healthy child with foreign proteins and toxic substances. [A recent study in *Lancet* (April 29, 1995, pp. 1071-1073) found that people who had received the measles vaccine were three times more likely to develop Crohn's disease and more than twice as likely to develop ulcerative colitis than people who did not receive the vaccine.]

Q. We very seldom know the long-term effects of any drug. There's always the potential for some sort of medicine that you took in the 1960s to have an effect on you in the 1990s.

NM: With one major difference: other drugs aren't mandatory. If you contract a disease and go to the hospital, you're entitled to accept or reject the doctor's recommended medicine, whether it's for you or your child. But the medical establishment and members of the government are lobbying to eliminate parental choice where childhood shots are concerned. They don't believe parents should be allowed to choose whether or not their children are vaccinated.

Q. Are these things going to show up in the child right away?

NM: The dangers associated with some vaccines are not always immediate. Just because your child didn't have an obvious reaction to the shots doesn't mean the vaccine was safe. There may be long-term effects. For example, in the 1950s and 1960s millions of people were inoculated with polio vaccines tainted with monkey viruses. At least one of those viruses, SV40, has been associated with new forms of cancer.[103]

Q. I've heard many horror stories over the pertussis vaccine. But are you saying there's also a latent effect with the other shots as well?

NM: This is certainly an important factor to consider. I've heard parents remark, "Our child was vaccinated and there were no problems." But post-vaccinal encephalitis — neurological damage — can occur following the shots even though an overt reaction wasn't observed.[104-109] How do you know whether your bright child with an IQ of 135 shouldn't have rightfully had an IQ of 145? How can we measure that? We just don't know the long-term consequences of injecting our healthy children with these foreign proteins and toxic substances.

Q. Somebody could argue that maybe they'd rather give up 10 percent of their IQ than contract the disease and perhaps die.

NM: The very reason parents should always have the freedom to choose whether or not to vaccinate their children.

Q. Maybe parents shouldn't be responsible for that decision because they could make the wrong one and injure the child.

NM: The government is neither willing nor able to take responsibility for a vaccine-damaged child. The vaccine decision must remain the parents' alone, especially when we consider all the conflicting studies on vaccines from around the world — valid studies that are often rejected without justification merely because the outcomes do not conform to the official stand held by the medical establishment.

Q. I'm a physician, and I don't dispute the idea that all parents should make informed decisions. But you made the statement that no one knows the long-term effects of injecting live viruses into children. That's deceptive, because as far as I know there

are no injectable live virus vaccines on the market.

NM: Many of the vaccines contain live viruses.

Q. But they're not injected. Only the oral polio vaccine has the live virus.

NM: That's not true.

Q. Name me another vaccine that's a live virus vaccine.

NM: Measles, mumps, rubella, some of the earlier Hib vaccines.

Q. I disagree with that. We have a difference of opinion.

NM: It's not a question of opinion, it's a question of fact. These vaccines contain live viruses. And some of the newer vaccines are genetically engineered.[110]

Q. At a recent annual American Cancer Society Science Writer Seminar, a university doctor warned that vaccination programs against flu, measles, mumps, and polio may actually be seeding humans with RNA that forms proviruses, which then become latent cells throughout the body. Activated, they can give rise to a variety of diseases, including chronic fatigue syndrome — also lupus, cancer, rheumatism, and arthritis.

NM: Again, many parents will think, "I took my child to the doctor for his shots and he didn't have a reaction, so everything is OK." But doctors are injecting our children with live viruses; they never leave the body. Instead, they fuse with healthy cells, which begin to replicate. Each succeeding mutation is one generation removed from a full, 100 percent healthy cell. And with each succeeding generation, the immune system apparently becomes more and more confused. It no longer knows if the virus that's been replicating with the healthy cells is something to repel or to leave alone. If it decides the compromised cells are foreign matter, and wages battle, we may be looking at new forms of cancer. If, instead, it chooses to disregard pleas for aid from the violated cells, and closes down its security measures, we may be risking an increase in autoimmune malfunctions and allergic responses.

Q. When these vaccines are injected, they are bypassing the body's natural defenses. Rather than going through the mouth, where you've got the tonsils, or through the nose, skin, and other natural defenses, the vaccine bypasses them.

NM: Most people don't realize how complex the immune system is. It comprises many different aspects of the human body. The medical establishment, however, has convinced us that antibody production is about the only immune system defense available, a clever ploy when you consider the vaccine is designed only to stimulate antibody production. Medical people do not give due credit to all the other immune system defenses responsible for maintaining a healthy organism.

Q. It's like saying, we need only soldiers to fight the enemy. We don't need ammunition, weapons, food and transportation.

NM: Right.

Q. I just read an article in the *New York Times* on a study published in the *British Medical Journal* confirming a thesis advanced in recent years by scientists in England that children exposed to infectious agents early in life may gain immunity to childhood leukemia and cancer of the blood. What this says to me is that it's important for children to get sick naturally, to develop these maladies, like measles and mumps, to immunize themselves naturally. Let the infectious agent go through its normal pathways: the nose, the ears, the throat, and the eyes, instead of not doing it.

NM: I agree. It appears that children who contract relatively minor diseases early on may be strengthening their immune systems to tackle more dangerous diseases later.[111]

Q. I'm a chiropractor, not a medical doctor, and so I concur heartily with everything you've said. None of my children have been vaccinated. I personally believe that the human genome, or the human family, has been compromised by injecting foreign proteins into our children. Could you please comment on the increase in juvenile leukemia, also the evidence of increased polio due to live polio vaccines being injected, and also some of the autoimmune collagen diseases that are now cropping up that I think may have a tie-in with the vaccines.

NM: Research indicates that when a vaccine is injected directly into the body, it bypasses normal immune system responses, and in so doing, sets up a number of conditions that can lead to protective malfunctions.[112] The various conditions you refer to are the possible results.

Q. So in effect we're trading off very common and relatively innocuous childhood diseases for more insidious ailments like

chronic fatigue syndrome and cancer.

NM: Exactly. Research indicates that by grappling with some of these childhood diseases, the immune system matures and is strengthened to fight future ailments.[113]

Q. I'm a pediatrician. There is no data to support that the vaccine virus being given had anything to do with changing the immune system down the road, or causing allergies, or promoting cancer. I've never seen any documented evidence. And I believe, if there were, we would be hard-pressed to justify giving the vaccine.

NM: A lot of very well-respected studies conducted throughout the world show correlations between the vaccines, the vaccine campaigns, and the breakdown of the immune system. For example, in 1975, when Japan raised the age to receive vaccines from two months to two years, the incidence of Sudden Infant Death Syndrome (SIDS) virtually disappeared in that country.[114] In 1991, the Institute of Medicine released a report documenting a causal relationship between the rubella vaccine and acute arthritis in adult women.[115] Links have also been found between this vaccine and chronic fatigue syndrome.[116] And in 1992, the World Health Organization suspended use of a new measles vaccine after realizing it was killing young children. Children who received the vaccine were dying in significantly greater numbers *from other diseases* than children who did not receive the vaccine. This indicates that this measles vaccine, and perhaps others like it, are capable of breaking down the immune system and allowing other diseases to occur. This vaccine was quietly withdrawn from the market.[117]

Q. Did they say it was because the children had preexisting conditions or were malnourished?

NM: No, because the death rate of children who received this vaccine was compared with that of similar children who did not receive the vaccine. The expected mortality of the young Africans in the study was estimated at 4 per 1,000 children at five months of age; the actual mortality was 75 per 1,000 children. The children were dying from a variety of common childhood illnesses. In fact, the authors of the study noted that previous studies suggest "the 'interaction' of live measles vaccines with child immunity is possible."[118]

Q. Is it true that elementary school teachers who taught before and after the introduction of mass vaccination programs have actually seen a decrease in children's learning abilities? Are the

intelligence tests given to children today easier than tests given to the same age groups before the vaccines were routinely administered?

NM: Beginning in the 1960s, soon after mass vaccination programs had started, both the average scores on standardized tests and the degree of difficulty of the tests fell consistently. It is estimated that the average schoolchild today is performing at levels up to two grades behind those of children who attended school before vaccination campaigns were initiated.[119]

Q. What about hyperactivity and various behavioral disorders? What does your research show in that regard?

NM: You may be referring to some very insightful research by Dr. Harris Coulter. He wrote a book, *Vaccination, Social Violence, and Criminality*, documenting correlations between mass vaccination programs, new diseases, and social ills.[120] He revealed correlations found between the pertussis vaccine and varying degrees of neurological damage.[121] There were no known cases of autism — a unique form of brain damage — anywhere in the world until after the pertussis vaccine was introduced.[122] Once mass vaccination programs were initiated, thousands of cases were diagnosed in the "developed" countries each year.[123-125] Today, 15 to 20 percent of all children in our school systems are diagnosed as learning disabled. Many of them have attention deficit hyperactivity disorder, or minimal brain dysfunction.[126-128] These are other conditions virtually unheard of before the advent of mass vaccination programs.

Q. Is it possible that it simply wasn't diagnosed, that the malady was there and was not recognized?

NM: When you go back and study the records, you'll find that these conditions simply weren't there in these numbers. Consider autism. This condition was unheard of — with or without a name — until 1943, soon after the pertussis vaccine was introduced. By the 1960s, soon after national vaccination campaigns were instituted, the condition began occurring in epidemic proportions.[129]

Q. Once the vaccine is put into the body, does it remain there forever, or is there a way for the body to throw it off, including the formaldehyde, mercury, and other toxic substances?

NM: Because a virus, upon entering the body, fuses with healthy cells and begins to replicate, many (but not all) health practitioners insist that the viral aspect of the vaccine, once injected, cannot be removed. I have been told, however, that a nutritional balance may be achieved, rendering the virus powerless. As for the mercury, formaldehyde, and other vaccine ingredients, I recommend consulting with a naturopathic or homeopathic health practitioner. Many have been trained to offer antidotes for toxic substances.

AIDS

Q. Do you think AIDS is connected to vaccinations?

NM: I think it's a significant line of inquiry. Plausible theories linking vaccines to AIDS have been considered. Some researchers believe AIDS started with polio vaccines that were tainted with monkey viruses.[130] Others think it was manmade and later tested on Central Africans during a smallpox vaccine campaign.[131] Still others link AIDS with early hepatitis B vaccine trials.[132]

Q. Were you aware that the AIDS virus is manmade? It was developed by the United States.

NM: I have copies of congressional records from 1969 in which the U.S. military sought funds for mixing viruses to create a germ that would affect the immune system.[133] [As revealed in _Immunization Theory vs. Reality,_ see page 79.] Is that what you're talking about?

Q. Yes. The project was code-named "N.K. Naomi." They developed the virus at Ft. Detrick, Maryland. Later, in San Francisco and New York, it was introduced in the hepatitis B vaccine. It was also used in Africa.

NM: This issue is huge, and we're only looking at the tip of the iceberg.

Q. Are you familiar with the Strecker Memorandum?

NM: Yes. In 1987 the _London Times_ published a story uncovering correlations between vaccines and a manmade AIDS virus said to have been created by United States scientists and tested on Central Africans.[134]

Q. In November I telephoned the county health department where I grew up and had received my smallpox and polio shots in 1957. I told the nurse I was working on my family medical history and asked if she'd send me a copy of my vaccine records. She told me they were no longer available — they had been destroyed. She gave me no explanation of how or why. I wonder if the vaccine records in other counties were destroyed

as well. If officials don't have any records, how are they going to confirm whether the vaccines lead to AIDS or anything else?

NM: Good observation. That might prove to be an interesting research project.

Q. My fear of vaccinating my children is that they might get the AIDS virus from the vaccine.

NM: Your fear is probably unfounded, but we do need to look at how often these vaccines are used on various populations to test theories that medical scientists and defense officials have devised.

Q. What do you think about a vaccine against AIDS?

NM: The worst possible thing scientists could do in seeking out a cure for AIDS is to come up with a vaccine against it.[135] AIDS already breaks down the immune system. I believe a vaccine for AIDS would hasten this process and place healthy people at risk as well.

Q. What's going to happen with AIDS if they don't come up with a vaccine or some way to control it?

NM: I don't have the answer to that, but I believe a vaccine won't solve the problem.

GOVERNMENT and LAWS

Q. The Clinton administration announced plans to implement a $1 billion program to vaccinate all United States children. Under this proposal, children would be required to receive vaccinations at the time of birth or shortly thereafter. An important feature of this proposal is the creation of a nationwide tracking system that would require all children to be registered at birth in a centralized computer databank. Provisions for a religious or philosophical exemption from mandatory vaccination would not be included in the bill. The law would be designed so that if a child does not show up to get a shot, bells and whistles will go off. The American Civil Liberties Union and groups advocating parental rights and vaccine safety are voicing concerns about this plan. It's very Orwellian.

NM: Congress and the President are tightening the grips around the American people. They are pushing to make vaccine laws more restrictive. At present, most states allow parents to object to the vaccines and still enter public school.[136] School officials rarely inform parents about these exemptions — personal, religious, and medical — yet you can sign a waiver. The new law, however, is set up to track parents who resist, and may seek to eliminate these exemptions.[137] Keep in mind that some lawmakers believe that if a parent refuses to vaccinate their child, even after having read the pros and cons, that parent should be charged with child abuse.

Q. You mean they'd have to do jail time?

NM: I know of parents whose unvaccinated children have been taken from them by court order.

Q. You mean this is happening even before the new bill has gone through?

NM: Absolutely. I recently received a call from a very distressed mother in California. Her three-year-old daughter had scraped her knee and had to be taken to the hospital emergency room. The nurses wanted to know if the child was up-to-date on her shots, and the woman said she was opposed to them. Even though California offers a very humane vaccine waiver law — opposition to the shots is permitted based on personal beliefs — the hospital contacted Social Services, which got in touch with the district attorney, who took the woman to court. The last I heard, the state was trying to gain custody of the child to force the injections on her. Hospital officials, Social Services, and the courts will often try to intimidate one family to scare others into vaccinating their children.

Q. This sounds like a Communist tactic.

NM: It is not as uncommon as you might think. Most people do not realize the battles that are being fought right now to preserve parental rights in this area.

Q. I've been trying to read between the lines of what President Clinton and Hillary are saying about childhood vaccinations. Is there anything that you're aware of in what they're proposing?

NM: They want to make vaccines universally accessible. They're proposing to allocate additional funds so that all U.S. children may receive the shots. But their propaganda is dishonest. For example, they claim that for every dollar we spend now, we'll save ten in the future.[138] But they conveniently forgot to factor into their figures, and deceitfully neglected to tell the American people, that more than $500 million has already been spent compensating parents for their children who were damaged or killed by the shots.[139]

Q. I guess a lot of lawyers make a pretty good living representing families of vaccine-damaged children.

NM: No, they don't. Congress put a cap on the amount of money that lawyers can make representing these cases.

Q. I don't believe in anything compulsory, and it would appear, from what I have heard so far, that the government is doing everything it can to take children away from their parents.

NM: You're absolutely right, and I feel exactly like you do, that if some parents elect to have their children vaccinated, fine. But the government also needs to respect the decisions of parents who choose against the vaccines.

Q. The Clinton definition of preventive health care is more mammography, drugs for senior citizens, and making sure everyone in the United States is vaccinated. What's your response to this?

NM: I'm getting reactions from all over the country. Parents are outraged that the government is attempting to mandate vaccines without looking at the specifics of each individual child.

Q. It concerns me that doctors will take the same vaccine and put it into every child at six weeks of age, when the immune system is not even fully developed, before they even know what kind of child this is, what kind of reactions the child may have. I know many people are never asked for a family history, drug allergies, anything like that. What is a parent to do?

NM: I recommend getting involved.

Q. We're talking about the government requiring these shots. I'm not going to have any say about whether I want them for my child. The government is saying we have to do it, we can't get our kids into school without it, and a federal registry will be set up to track parents who resist, something we still don't do with child abusers. The government is going to exchange information about whether or not our kids have their shots. This isn't right.

NM: I agree. Some of the other bills that are being proposed right now include the allocation of money for the development of what is described as a "supervaccine," and a proposal designed to deny welfare benefits to parents who refuse the shots.[140,141] The supervaccine is simply mad science. Medical authorities want to stick a swarm of time-released viruses into one shot so that parents won't have to make extra trips to the clinic.[142]

Q. Looking at these bills, what are your thoughts? Are they going to go through?

NM: I think these bills will pass because all the cards are stacked in the proponents' favor. For example, at a recent so-called public meeting on this issue, authorities invited Donna Shalala, secretary of Health and Human Services; Marion Wright Edelman, director of the Children's Defense Fund; presidents of four companies that produce vaccines; representatives of the American Academy of Pediatrics; and public health officials. But they would not allow representatives from the National Vaccine Information Center — a national organization particularly concerned about vaccine safety — to attend.[143]

Q. Mr. Miller, without your book how would any of us know about these problems? Who's been derelict? Who, if anyone, has been negligent? Where has the media been? Has everyone sort of been asleep?

NM: In 1986, the U.S. government finally acknowledged that vaccine-induced damage and death was occurring, and in large numbers. Congress enacted a law that would permit families of vaccine-damaged children to be compensated. Most people do not realize that when they go to the pediatrician's office to have their children vaccinated, they are paying a tax on every vaccine they buy. The money goes into a congressional fund to pay for children who are damaged.

Q. What else does this law require?

NM: Doctors must report vaccine reactions. However, many refuse to comply by simply denying that a reaction occurred, even though a mother or a father may have voiced such concerns.[144]

Q. The government says that only 40 to 60 percent of preschool children get their recommended shots. Some diseases are showing up again, and one of the reasons is because people just can't afford it. In 1982 you could have gotten the full battery of shots for $23. In 1992, the cost was $244 — a tenfold increase. This is why the Clinton administration proposed a nationwide vaccine registry. It would help doctors and local officials identify preschool children who have a high risk of illness because they did not get the recommended vaccines.

NM: Every time a parent buys a vaccine, a large portion of the cost of the vaccine goes into a special congressional fund to compensate the percentage of children authorities know will be brain-damaged or die from the vaccine. This is one of the reasons for the 1,000 percent increase in the price of vaccines.

Q. The additional fee is only about two dollars per vaccine.

NM: The government has already spent more than $500 million just in the past few years compensating families of victims.[145]

Q. I understand that the compensation situation had to do with the degree of litigiousness in society, which was preventing people from getting their children adequately immunized. It was to take it out of the medical spheres allowing people who have experienced some of the side effects to be compensated when they appear to have been due to vaccination.

NM: National TV just uncovered a government scandal related to the compensation system. Evidently, when a child dies from the vaccine, the government is only liable for $250,000, but if the child lives and requires lifetime care, awards can go as high as $3 or $4 million. So officials drag these cases on hoping the child will pass away. Moreover, recent FDA figures acknowledge more than 34,000 adverse reactions to vaccines, including nearly 700 deaths, in just the last three and a half years ending January 1994.[146] The true figures could be much higher because the FDA admits that 90 percent of doctors refuse to report such incidents.[147] Yet, these cases are not examined. The government is either so indifferent to the possibility that vaccine damage is epidemic in our society, or so afraid of opening Pandora's box, that it refuses to investigate or follow up on these cases. They're not interested in looking at these children, or talking with their parents. This is why I am warning parents; the government doesn't care. It doesn't want you to hear what I have to say. And neither does the medical establishment. They just want to keep the whole issue quiet. Maintaining the status quo is more important to them than warning parents to beware or to look into the issue, or than investigating the true extent of vaccine damage.

Q. I'm from Illinois, and our state has required a nine-page flyer on each vaccine be given to parents when they choose to have their child receive a shot. Do you know if this is a national law?

NM: Yes, it is. In 1986, Congress enacted this law, requiring parents to read about the potential risks associated with vaccines before agreeing to the shots. In my opinion, these booklets are inadequate. They discount the true dangers, and seem designed instead to frighten parents into vaccinating their children.[148]

Q. I am a pediatrician, and I think it's a valid requirement to have all children immunized. In the minds of a significant number of experts, vaccines are protective for those children who receive them. And there is a public health issue here as well. Children with communicable diseases, in the early stages when they're most communicable, have the potential for effect on the children obviously in danger, because they're in school together. Therefore, children, if allowed to be vulnerable to infectious disease, will communicate it if they're not protected through a vaccine. So it's an individual child measure and it's a public health measure as well, which are both good rationales in my mind.

NM: Children who are not vaccinated cannot be a health threat to children who are vaccinated if the vaccines are effective.

Q. I am a natural health practitioner, and I think that drug companies have to charge so much because people are getting hurt as a result of the amount of drugs we're using on our population, causing lawyers to become involved. Drug companies have so much product liability going on that in order to offset what they're going to lose as a result of damaging people, they have to charge more.

NM: From the 1980s to the 1990s, the price of vaccines increased by 1,000 percent.[149] A large reason for this is that the vaccine manufacturers were being sued, and they compensated for the money they were losing in those lawsuits by raising the prices.[150]

Q. The drug companies are steadily expanding their employee base and their manufacturing. In fact, as the _Physicians' Desk Reference_, the _PDR_, gets thicker, we as a nation get sicker. We don't spend enough time and money considering preventive health measures, so of course that industry is doing well. But if the drug companies were doing such a great job and were helping humanity so much, why are we getting sicker?

NM: That's a good question.

STATE WAIVERS

Q. I heard that you can't get unvaccinated children into some schools. I also heard that children can be exempt from the shots if their parents have strong feelings against them. How does that work? What are the legal requirements?

NM: Many doctors and school officials try to convince parents that the vaccines are mandatory. Authorities may even threaten to bar your child from entering school. Every state, however, offers one or more exemptions to the vaccines, based on your religious convictions, personal beliefs, or your child's medical contraindications.[151] Officials are currently putting pressure on state lawmakers to remove these options — "loopholes" to authorities — from the books. I consider this a wicked and immoral endeavor, because parents are entitled to full disclosure of the facts and freedom of choice. Contact your state health department to find out the exact requirements. Or go to the library and obtain a copy of the vaccine laws of your state. In many cases, exempting your child is as simple as signing a form indicating that you object to the vaccines. [For more information on how you can obtain the exact laws of your state, turn to pages 79 and 80.]

Q. In the old days, without that smallpox vaccination, our kids literally couldn't get into first grade. I guess that was before passage of the exemptions.

NM: It's not very different today.

Q. What do you mean?

NM: I receive many calls and letters from distressed parents who are threatened and blackmailed by school officials.

Q. But when they stand up to the school officials and say, "I don't want my child vaccinated. Here's the form that I've prepared and signed showing why I don't want my child vaccinated," then the school official has to back down. Is that right?

NM: In theory, that's correct. But I've observed that if you're a weak-willed parent, or waver on the issue, authorities will smell blood and stay on the attack.

Q. You're right. I remember getting notes from my kids' school, years ago, saying, "We don't have your child's vaccination records. If they are not here by Tuesday at noon, your child will not be allowed in school on Wednesday." Nowhere did

it say, "unless you come up with a declaration showing that you refuse to give your kids the shots."

NM: There's a lot of hostility toward parents who refuse vaccines.

Q. Maybe there is a fear that parents are unwittingly subjecting their children to potential harm.

NM: This confirms my belief that everyone needs to be better informed.

Q. I'm a concerned parent, and I want to do the proper thing for my children. How do I deal with the pressure? I mean, if my child can't get in school, then what have I accomplished?

NM: First, decide if you're for or against vaccines. Then, be firm in your convictions. If you don't want your child vaccinated, sign the form, have it notarized, and give it to the school nurse.

Q. I would be willing to bet that the public health department won't tell me how to do that.

NM: That's probably a good bet. School nurses and the principal may oppose you as well. But that shouldn't stop you from doing what you believe is best for your child.

Q. The school nurse said that if my child doesn't get vaccinated and then gets the disease, he'll give it to the other children.

NM: That argument doesn't make sense. In fact, it bolsters the argument _against_ vaccinations. If the other children are vaccinated, and the vaccines work, how can those children be susceptible to your child's illness?

Q. If parents have the right to object to vaccines, is the school liable when a child becomes ill with a virus that may have been spread at school?

NM: No. When a parent signs the waiver objecting to vaccines, the parent remains responsible if the child contracts a disease.

Q. In order to get into some colleges, students are required to be vaccinated. It seems that we're getting vaccinated for the wrong reasons.

NM: Yes, students are reporting that college administrators are trying to force them into receiving the shots prior to admission, just as the federal government is trying to force welfare recipients into vaccinating their children in order to keep receiving benefits.[152]

THEORY vs. REALITY

Q. What is the principle behind vaccines?

NM: That if you take a weakened form of a virus that would normally give you a disease, and inject it into the body, disease-fighting antibodies will be produced.

Q. But those antibodies may only be fighting what was injected into the body, including chemicals and other substances.

NM: Good observation. Nevertheless, if antibodies against the injection are produced, the vaccine is considered effective.

Q. Do vaccines work? If it was evident that they don't work, we wouldn't have to worry about side effects. If officials have us asking the wrong questions, they don't have to worry about the answers. According to your research, how does it stack up?

NM: The evidence indicates that vaccine efficacy rates are dismal.[153-157] In fact, double-blind studies — the gold standard of scientific research — are rarely conducted within the vaccine community.

Q. That's what authorities are demanding from chiropractors. Yet, when medical scientists grope for the truth, they call it a clinical study. When anyone else conducts research, they call it anecdotal.

NM: Such ploys are common.

Q. Are any of the shots capable of eradicating disease?

NM: I doubt it. Prior to smallpox vaccination campaigns, smallpox circulated throughout society, whereas today it ceases to exist. The medical establishment claims there is a connection, even though the evidence indicates that smallpox epidemics ended after people began *refusing* the shots. On the other hand, prior to smallpox vaccination campaigns, cancer didn't occur in epidemic numbers, autism didn't exist, and hyperactivity and autoimmune ailments were barely known. Now the medical establishment claims there is *not* a connection. This double standard of scientific conduct has fooled countless numbers of otherwise very bright people.

Q. Do you believe the antibody premise is a flawed premise altogether, and that there isn't a single vaccination that's good for somebody to get? Or are you just questioning whether or not everyone should be vaccinated?

NM: I don't recommend for or against the vaccines. I advocate freedom of choice. This right should never be taken from a parent. That said, I believe the antibody premise is flawed for several reasons. First, antibody production does not guarantee disease prevention. This has been proven again and again. Blood serum tests may indicate that the individual is "protected," yet the disease may still be contracted. Conversely, there are many instances of low or nonexistent antibody levels in "unprotected" people who are later exposed to the disease and don't get it. Second, the ability to stimulate antibodies is a neat trick, but the immune system is more complex than this. Diseased matter injected directly into the body dangerously bypasses the entire network of defensive measures normally available to fight infection. Third, the vaccines contain toxic substances, a potentially fatal flaw considering our current knowledge of mercury, aluminum, and formaldehyde. Finally, the unknown long-term effects of tampering with the delicate human immune system dictates a more cautious approach.

RISKS vs. BENEFITS

Q. Isn't it a greater risk to get one of the childhood diseases than to get the vaccine itself?

NM: I don't think so, but if you say it enough times, people will start believing it — evidence that even if vaccines aren't effective, medical propaganda is.

Q. But the vaccines are supposed to empower the immune system to fight off the diseases.

NM: The vaccines are produced by companies that have a financial stake in continuing to produce them. This cannot be overlooked. We'd all like to believe that the motivations of the medical establishment and pharmaceutical companies are 100 percent altruistic. I'm asking parents to wake up. We need to look into this matter and realize that vaccination is a very lucrative business. These people are extremely interested in seeing that your child is vaccinated, but not necessarily for the reasons you'd like to believe.

Q. How many people are hurt each year by the vaccines?

NM: Some researchers estimate the true figure to be several thousand per year in the United States alone, especially if you consider many of the cases of minimal brain damage, learning disabilities, and hyperactivity disorder.[158]

Q. Which children are most at risk?

NM: The American Academy of Pediatrics (AAP) has a list of the types of children who should not receive vaccines.[159] But has your pediatrician ever questioned you to determine if vaccinating your child is contraindicated? Probably not. Doctors simply administer the shots. But some children are at a greater risk for vaccine damage than others. You need to find out whether your child is a high-risk child. Ask your pediatrician for a copy of the AAP vaccine contraindications. Ask to see the warnings published by the vaccine makers as well. I guarantee this will annoy your doctor, and he or she may even refuse your request, but you're the one who is ultimately responsible for your child's care.

Q. I don't know if I'm all that capable of deciphering and evaluating the risks and benefits of taking vaccines.

NM: You have the choice of continuing to follow the standard recommendations without question, or of researching this matter further until you are satisfied that you are making a wise decision, whatever it may be.

Q. What are some of the side effects of the vaccines?

NM: The following conditions have each been investigated as a consequence of, or have been scientifically confirmed as resulting from, one or more of the vaccines: fever, rashes, itching, bruises, headache, pain, soreness, sore throat, inflamed sinuses, swelling, diarrhea, projectile vomiting, excessive sleepiness, inconsolable crying, high-pitched screaming, tics, tremors, seizures, collapse, convulsions, anaphylactic shock, loss of consciousness, breathing problems, cranial nerve palsies, encephalitis, grand mal epilepsy, neurological disorders, weak muscles, paralysis, polio, aseptic meningitis, epiglottitis, multiple sclerosis, Reye's syndrome, Guillain-Barré syndrome, chronic fatigue syndrome, Sudden Infant Death Syndrome (SIDS), blood-clotting disorders, urinary and abdominal complications, juvenile-onset diabetes, pneumonia, liver abnormalities, arthralgia, rheumatoid arthritis, unilateral nerve deafness, polyneuritis, measles, atypical measles, pertussis, mumps, meningitis, inner-ear nerve damage, recurrent abscess formation, demyelinating neuropathy, EEG abnormalities, dyslexia, visual defects, hearing loss, speech impediments, T-lymphocyte blood count reductions, haemophilus influenzae, influenza, small-pox, AIDS, cancer, leukemia, lupus erythematosus, genetic muta-tions, autoimmune disorders, autism, childhood schizophrenia, brain tumors, developmental disabilities, learning disorders, hyper-activity disorder, juvenile delinquency, drug abuse, alcoholism, violent crime, mental retardation, brain damage, and death.[159]

Q. Many people assume the vaccines _are_ safe and effective. If they weren't, the government wouldn't want everybody to be vaccinated, right?

NM: That's the assumption. But has the government ever been wrong? The Department of Energy recently released a report detail-ing the government's willing involvement in radioactive tests on human beings.[161] When people get around to uncovering the vaccine scandal, I guarantee it will make other issues pale in comparison.

Q. Everything has a risk, though, even tap water. Where do we draw the line between acceptable and unacceptable risk?

NM: Everything may have a risk, but everything isn't mandatory. If these vaccines have the potential to be dangerous, and are known to be ineffective, then it is unconscionable to mandate them.

Q. You talk about the long-term effects, but the immediate effects concern me. Children get their shots, are rushed to the morgue, and yet their pediatricians say the two events are not related. Or they exhibit a variety of symptoms that, if they arose under different circumstances, would prompt any parent to rush them to an emergency room. But doctors tell parents it's just a normal response to the vaccine.

NM: There's a remarkable fellowship among medical associates. Initiation into the club required a large financial commitment and many grueling years of difficult study. Now, doctors are terrified of speaking out or of breaking rank. The perceived penalties are too great.

Q. Dr. Robert Mendelsohn once told me that less than 50 percent of pediatricians in this country vaccinate their own children. They are worried about reactions. They would rather give vaccines to their patients than to their own children.

NM: I often wonder how these doctors can sleep at night.

Q. My child is almost nine years old, and she's never had any of the vaccines. Is it less safe for her to get them now, or is this

just a back-and-forth quandary? Do you have any suggestions?

NM: The pertussis vaccine is not given to children after the age of seven because it is especially dangerous beyond that point, although a lot of research indicates it can be quite dangerous before that point as well. The measles vaccine is now being given to high school and college students. You're just going to have to weigh the evidence and make your decision.

Q. What would you consider the risks to be if you've had a child with a reaction?

NM: I would consider them to be high. There may be a genetic factor; certain families may be more susceptible to the dangers of the vaccines. It's something to consider, and I think you have a responsibility to look into it further.

Q. Say a child had the initial round of these vaccines *without* any adverse reactions or with minor reactions like redness, soreness, and fever, and another shot is required at 14 years of age. Does it mean the child will be much less likely to have a severe reaction, having weathered the first round fairly well?

NM: No. It means the vaccines are ineffective, and instead of coming out and being honest with you by saying, "We're sorry, but our vaccines are ineffective," the authorities are saying, "Line up again, we want to give your child more of our ineffective vaccines."

Q. Do you believe the risks are unacceptable for all vaccines? Should a parent never have a child vaccinated?

NM: That's a personal decision. I simply offer a warning that vaccines may be unsafe and ineffective. When you consider all the contrary studies that the medical establishment and government officials don't want you to know about, it becomes ever more clear that parents have an obligation to investigate the issue. And their right to choose against vaccinating their children must be maintained.

PERSONAL STORIES

Q. I have a nine-year-old niece who was vaccinated with MMR in order to get into school. Now she's in Children's Hospital going through all sorts of tests and physical therapies. She can't walk or talk, and the doctors can't figure out what's wrong.

NM: I'm very sorry to hear that. Sadly, I get calls like yours all the time, and letters too, from parents, friends, and concerned relatives of children who were perfectly healthy until they received the shots.

Q. She was perfectly healthy.

NM: And now these children are either brain-damaged or dead.

Q. A couple I know had their baby at the hospital. The doctors knew the parents didn't want the shots for their baby, but the first thing they tried to do when the baby was born was give the shots. The dad had to raise a pretty big stink to have them withhold the shots.

NM: Intimidation tactics by medical personnel are very common.

Q. But he had to get almost physical before they backed off.

NM: This is why I recommend that parents remain clear about the choices they make and stand firm in their convictions.

Q. I agree that parents need to make choices. My eight-year-old daughter is severely disabled due to a vaccine-related injury. I'm one of those parents who has a compensation suit from the federal government for MMR. I just want to say that I think we need to be able to make choices and decide on our own what we want to do about vaccinating our kids. I chose not to vaccinate my other children as a result of her severe disabilities. She cannot walk or talk, must be fed, dressed, and cared for by a nurse's aide. We're talking about a *severe* disability.

NM: I'm sorry to hear that. Did your pediatrician inform you of the potential dangers before your child was given the shots?

Q. No. Our daughter had been vaccinated in the regular series up to 18 months. She was supposed to have a 15-month MMR shot along with DPT at 18 months. So I took her in at 18 months and they gave her all six of them together.

NM: I'm very sorry. I just received a call from a woman whose child became autistic after being inoculated with the MMR vaccine. She spends 24 hours a day caring for her child, but she will not be compensated by the fund. The government comes up with all sorts of technicalities to avoid helping these families.

Q. We can't even get the physicians to say that's actually what's

wrong, although they cannot find any other reason for the severity of the illness. Imagine taking a normal, healthy child and having this happen.

NM: There are absolutely no studies on giving children what your child received, six vaccine mixtures at once. Yet, doctors are taking our healthy children and shooting them up with combination vaccines. I'll tell you why. It has nothing to do with whether or not it's a safe procedure; it's a marketing ploy. Doctors are concerned that if parents have to make several trips for the vaccines, they're not going to do it. So they figure, "Since we already have them in the office, let's shoot 'em up with several vaccines at once."[162]

Q. You scare new parents whose relatives are saying, "You have to get the shots." Now we hear the child could be seriously injured or die.

NM: How many times has the government said one thing, and then years later we found out something different? We learn that pregnant mothers have been taking this or that drug and it's hurt their children, even though it was sanctioned by the government. Or we find that Agent Orange hurt our service troops, even though the government denied that it could cause problems. That's all I'm saying. I know some parents are going to be a little bit scared, but, again, all I'm trying to do is wake people up to look into the issue. And if you've got a newborn baby, now is the time to look into it.

Q. I really want to encourage you to continue your campaign to enlighten people on the dangers of vaccines. I happen to be one of the unlucky ones. I have a little boy who was damaged by the DPT shot when he was six months old.

NM: I'm sorry about your son. What is the nature of the damage?

Q: It's a broad range of many things. He's been diagnosed as mildly retarded, with hyperactivity, attention-deficit disorder, and learning and developmental disabilities.

NM: Has it been ascertained officially that the vaccine was the cause of this?

Q. Yes, it has, as a matter of fact, and it struck a chord when you were talking about the government dragging out their cases, because a year ago this past October we had our court case, our hearing, and it was determined that the pertussis vaccine did cause all his problems, but we're still waiting to be compensated.

NM: Did you have to hire an attorney?

Q. Yes, and our hearing was over the phone.

NM: There are so many cases that you can do this over the phone?

Q. I don't know all the statistics, but our particular case was done over the telephone, before a "grandmaster." Basically, he's the judge. The government has a lawyer, and we have a lawyer. Everyone presents testimony and evidence.

NM: In your particular case, the dangers definitely outweighed the benefits. I'm sorry you had to learn this the hard way.

Q. I wish I would have known before I gave my son the vaccines all that I know now. That's what I really wanted to say. You're doing a great job. You're not scaring parents. You just need to keep telling parents to get informed before they have their kids vaccinated. I say the same thing to people who meet my son and want to know about him and what happened. I just tell them. I don't ever tell anyone not to have their child vaccinated. I just tell them to get informed, read about it before doing anything, and then make an informed decision.

NM: Thanks for your input.

Q. I have seven children, and nineteen grandchildren. I was born in the late '30s, and grew up in the '40s and '50s when there were no vaccines. I have sympathy for the parents whose children were damaged by the vaccines, and maybe they shouldn't have been vaccinated when the child had a cold. But are we going to go back to quarantines, where the public health department nails a sign on the door and says you can't leave for two weeks? Are we going to watch children choke to death from diphtheria or whooping cough? What about the damage that measles caused? And are we going to isolate everyone in the months of July, August, and early September as we did in the days of polio, because it was too terrifying to take our children to the grocery store and church?

NM: When did scientists come out with a scarlet fever vaccine?

Q. I don't know if they did.

NM: They didn't. What happened to that disease? The incidence of scarlet fever declined.

Q. What does that mean?

NM: It means that some of these diseases declined on their own. When they hit a virgin population the complication and fatality rates may be high. Once the population gains a herd immunity, then the disease becomes relatively innocuous. It may even disappear. For example, lets look at polio and scarlet fever. There were epidemics of polio, scientists came out with a polio vaccine, and now we rarely hear about this disease. The vaccine gets credited with its eradication. But there were also epidemics of scarlet fever. Although no scarlet fever vaccine was ever developed, this disease declined as well. How did that happen without a vaccine? We could also look at the plague. There was never a vaccine for this killer disease, yet it has virtually disappeared as well. So there are a lot of other factors that need to be considered.

Q. When my first child was born, I said to my pediatrician, a certified neonatologist, "I want the serum number on this pertussis vaccine." He looked at me in surprise and said, "Why?" And I said, "I have no intention of suing you because you're doing what you have to do. But my understanding is that the drug companies that are producing this vaccine have had an opportunity to produce safer vaccines, and have opted not to do this. I certainly would sue a drug company if need be. I spent too many years [as a teacher] in Special Education." From that point on, he automatically gave me the serum number. And it was very interesting because he said to me, "I want you to know that if your child has a reaction the first time he's given the vaccine, the likelihood of complications will increase with each dose thereafter."

NM: He was surprisingly frank.

Q. I have a grandson who's seven years old. He was recently diagnosed with a deficit disorder. What shots could have caused, or amplified, his condition?

NM: The pertussis vaccine appears to have the most potential for damage, but some researchers believe many of the vaccines are capable of causing neurological disorders.

Q. How can parents and grandparents undo the damage?

NM: I suggest consulting with a holistic health practitioner — a professionally trained naturopath or homeopath, for example. They are likely to be aware of the most promising corrective measures.

Q. I know a couple with a baby who had the shots and is now severely dysfunctional. They're having a hard time proving it, with the doctor and his lawyer denying it. It just ruined their lives.

NM: Not uncommon.

Q. I'm a registered nurse, and I've been concerned about vaccines for a number of years. I was influenced by Dr. Robert Mendelsohn, a pediatrician who taught pediatric interns at the University of Illinois. He agreed that vaccinations are dangerous and that the medical establishment is not telling us the truth. What I wanted to ask was, is it true that vaccinations have not been mandatory in Canada and some of the European countries, and that the incidence of these diseases has gone down in those countries?

NM: Yes. For example, when the United States mandated the polio vaccine, many European countries permitted freedom of choice, and yet polio epidemics ended in those countries as well.[163]

Q. My wife and I read a book by Dr. Mendelsohn, who talks about not giving the vaccinations. When our second child came along we decided not to give her the shots, and we also stopped giving them to our son. The doctors told us we wouldn't be able to get our children into school. We talked to some other parents who had done the same thing and found out that if you sign a waiver taking all the risk off the school, that you could put your child in the school. When we told our pediatrician, she said she was deciding whether she was going to stop seeing our children if they were not vaccinated. When my wife told her about our concerns, and shared with her the information that we had read, and explained why we didn't want to get the shots, she said that it was all just a bunch of nonsense, and that we were being stupid.

NM: I hear that all the time. I heard two similar accounts last week. When parents refused the vaccines, the pediatrician said, "Don't return, I don't want you back."

Q. We had to quit the pediatrician just for that reason.

NM: You have to find somebody you can trust.

Q. I know people who were turned away from their family physician for not allowing their children to be vaccinated. There is pressure coming at parents from all sides to go ahead and give their children the shots. What would you recommend?

NM: The medical establishment supports the loss of parental rights on this issue. Mothers and fathers should be thankful that they're no longer using the services of arrogant doctors who couldn't care less about their concerns.

Q. Our children don't get shots, but there's tremendous resentment from other parents. They're afraid our children will spread disease.

NM: That is an irrational fear and a bogus argument perpetuated by medical personnel and health officials. If the vaccines are effective, your unvaccinated children cannot be a threat to children who received the shots.

Q. The CDC is now claiming that there are a small number of people who cannot be vaccinated, because of severe allergies to vaccine ingredients, for example, and because of a small percentage of vaccine failures. They argue that these people are susceptible to disease, and their *only* hope of protection is that people around them are immune and cannot pass disease along to them.

NM: First of all, forcing *everyone* to be vaccinated is immoral, regardless of the rationale. Second, where is the *proof* that forcing everyone to be vaccinated is the *only* hope of protection for the 'small number of people' who cannot take vaccines? Third, this argument is a dishonest attempt to manipulate the masses with guilt by making people feel responsible for others' sickness. Politicians used this ploy after the Oklahoma bombing in an attempt to link groups they opposed to the actual bombing. Finally, consider the plausibility of a similar argument: Because violent crime is rampant throughout society, *everyone* must remain armed at all times. Everyone must carry a loaded pistol, and be able to show proof of having taken an advanced course in martial arts. This mandate is being made to protect yourself, *and to protect the 'small number of people' who cannot protect themselves* (because of missing fingers that cannot pull the trigger, for example), and because of the small percentage of gun failures. Would you agree with this campaign? Mind control, body control. Who has authority over how people elect to achieve health? Who has authority over what goes into our bodies and into the bodies of our children? The CDC? The FDA? The U.S. government? Or you and I and the people being affected?

Q. I think parents have the right to know what goes into their child's body. Doctors have an obligation to tell us.

NM: I agree. But since doctors won't tell you, you have an obligation to find out on your own.

Q. I have five children who were not vaccinated. They're very healthy. Their vaccinated friends, meanwhile, have all kinds of health problems. I can't help but believe that some of this illness has to do with the shots they received.

NM: A likely explanation.

Q. I have five children. The oldest three were vaccinated with all the required shots, and my oldest boy still brought whooping cough home. So they all five got it even though the oldest three were vaccinated against it. My brother-in-law entered the military two years later, and had an emergency liver transplant because the stuff in the vaccines they gave him destroyed his liver. I find it interesting that now, two years after Desert Storm, many of those vets are reporting a variety of health problems.

NM: That's right. I just want to repeat your story for clarification. Your oldest son was vaccinated against whooping cough, and yet he still contracted whooping cough and passed it on to his siblings, two of them having been vaccinated against it as well. That's very common. Several studies indicate that of all the cases of pertussis, around half of them are in vaccinated people.[164-171] About Desert Storm, Congress is considering how to help all of the many vets who returned from the Gulf War with "mysterious ailments" that may be attributed to the experimental vaccines they were injected with.[172,173] [Documented in _Immunization Theory vs. Reality_, p. 79.]

Q. My kids do real well without the shots. We believe strongly that the health of the host organism determines whether or not a person will come down with a disease. When I was a medic in Vietnam, I used to write off my own shot records. I never took any of the stupid shots. And yet we'd administer the shots to the guys who didn't ask us to just write them off. And lo and behold, those poor guys would get sicker than we would.

NM: I'm glad you found a way to protect yourself.

Q. I had planned not to give my children the vaccinations because I think it is stupid to inject them with the diseases, but at the time when one of my children was due to be injected, I was falsely accused of child abuse, so I was afraid Protective Services would take my kids away if I didn't do it.

NM: You're probably right. If you had refused to vaccinate your children at that time, the state probably would have used that as a strike against you.

Q. What do you recommend?

NM: I recommend that parents wake up and start looking at the facts. Lawmakers and the medical establishment are trying to take away your rights. Find ways to protect your children.

Q. I have three boys, and they're fine. They got all the shots. But this is the '90s. Isn't the whole vaccination thing outdated?

NM: I believe vaccinations were outdated 200 years ago when they were first conceived — outdated, uncivilized, mad, genocidal superstitions.

Q. I think vaccinations are a cheap investment for established medicine. Consider all the money that can be generated in the future from the many diseases that will be created, and all the drugs that will be bought.

NM: Are you suggesting the shots are creating a whole new crop of diseases that will keep the medical establishment in business?

Q. That's right.

NM: Possibly more out of ignorance than knowing, although the compulsory aspect of the shots makes me wonder. I perceive it as medical enslavement.

Q. And then everyone goes back to the doctor to get more drugs and antibiotics that keep the cycle going.

NM: Astute observation.

Q: Vaccines were generated by the drug companies. What a windfall when you get a mandated vaccine, a law requiring people to use your product.

NM: And now the manufacturers are exempt from liability. The government took over the responsibility for compensating victims. A major incentive toward improving dangerous vaccines has been removed.

Q. I'm not against vaccinations. I'm against forced, mandated, routine injections of every single person. That's what I'm

against — not having the freedom of choice.

NM: I agree.

Q. I don't think that people should be bullied into getting the vaccines. It's a personal choice. If you decide to do it, fine. If you don't, you should have the right to decide that.

NM: I agree.

Q. I disagree with vaccinations. I think a lot goes unreported by doctors.

NM: Reactions?

Q. Yes, because they wouldn't want to scare parents. I think a lot is reported as Sudden Infant Death Syndrome, and other things like that.

NM: The FDA recently admitted that 90 percent of doctors refuse to report adverse reactions.[174]

Q. I also think a lot of parents are afraid that if they don't give their children the vaccines, they will be unprotected against disease and disaster. Please comment on how we can maintain our children's health.

NM: There are health alternatives to be considered. Many parents still don't realize that breastfeeding their newborns is the best way to stimulate their babies' immune systems, getting them off to a great start in life.[175-177] Parents might also investigate homeopathic and naturopathic options before making their _informed_ decisions. Healthcare practitioners who practice these forms of treatment have, like their allopathic counterparts, spent many grueling years in accredited university programs studying the human body and other principles of well-being.

ADDITIONAL COMMENTS and CONCERNS

Q. Why, within the last few years, have we seen this assault on vaccines? As I see it, it's all part of a campaign opposed to established medicine, and it seems to be coming from people who are advocates of natural healing. Am I anywhere close to being right on this?

NM: I think that's a good assessment. People are tired of being treated without dignity, and they're mistrustful of the allopathic drug approach. This translates into more and more people deciding to take charge of their own health and the health of their loved ones. Alternative health options await their awakenings.

Q. Doesn't it stand to reason that healthcare, like any arena involving a lot of people who are highly emotional and searching for solutions, has a tendency to attract a lot of charlatans? If someone's been diagnosed with pancreatic or liver cancer, and, having given up on conventional care, is seeing somebody who will administer coffee enemas, doesn't that increase the person's risk of dying?

NM: The medical establishment does not own our health. Parents and legal guardians are entitled to complete freedom of choice. People are able to make rational decisions on their own.

Q. Is this what the campaign against vaccinations is all about — freedom of choice?

NM: I think it is. That's the main issue. How can we assess the true facts behind it all, and determine whether the vaccines are actually helping or hurting, if the medical establishment continues to lobby against parental freedom of choice?

Q. Seat belts save lives and so do vaccines. I think parents are being irresponsible if they don't vaccinate their children. You should go with the odds.

NM: We all want what's best for our children. Those who choose against the vaccines believe they are going with the odds. I think parents are being irresponsible if they refuse to investigate the vaccine dilemma before making their decisions.

Q. Do you think kids would be better off without vaccines?

NM: Many dangers have been associated with vaccines. Giving them may pose more risks than not giving them. But I never recommend for or against the shots. I sincerely believe parents need to make that decision on their own.

Q. Isn't it the case that with any drug or any other method of medical treatment, there are risks and benefits, there is a risk-versus-benefit ratio? Any time you inject somebody with a foreign substance, whether it's aspirin or pertussis or anything else, there are dangers involved.

NM: That may be true, but drugs are not mandatory. And we have to look at whether the true extent of the potential damage associated with vaccines is being revealed. I don't believe it is.

Q. In what respect?

NM: The American people remain unaware of the true extent of vaccine-related damage that has been acknowledged by Congress. This doesn't even come close to the extent of damage that goes unreported. The FDA admits that doctors are refusing to report adverse reactions to the shots, even though they are required to do so by law.

Q. How is that different from any other drug reaction? When a doctor sees a bad reaction in a patient given penicillin, does that doctor necessarily call the CDC or the FDA and report that as an adverse reaction?

NM: There's a big difference: doctors are required by federal law to communicate vaccine reactions to a central reporting agency. But when parents discuss their child's violent response to the shot with their doctor, the doctor evades the law by simply denying that it was a reaction to the vaccine.

Q. Have we all been duped?

NM: I believe we have been. The medical establishment is a large and powerful organization. It influences the research institutions responsible for conducting the "unbiased" vaccine studies, the government officials responsible for drafting the laws, and the media responsible for shaping public opinion.

Q. Do you think the media and the medical profession try to scare the public into vaccinating their children?

NM: The media merely relays to the public the information they are supplied with by the medical establishment. Scare tactics — and outright lies — are common ploys used by the medical corps.

Q. I remember getting shots for polio, measles, and tetanus. What are doctors giving shots for today?

NM: If you follow medical recommendations, by the time your child reaches a few years of age, he or she will have received nearly 20 vaccines, totaling more than 30 injected or ingested germs and other toxic substances. The DPT and MMR vaccines contain disgusting matter from three diseases. The full battery of vaccines includes two MMRs, five DPTs, four oral polios, four Hibs, and three hepatitis B vaccines. The chickenpox vaccine is expected to be licensed for use, and mandated for all children, very soon as well. [On March 17, 1995, the FDA announced that it had approved the chickenpox vaccine. Shortly thereafter, the American Academy of Pediatrics began recommending it for all infants.] And the "magic bullet supervaccine," expected to contain numerous time-released germs, may be just around the corner.

Q. Please comment on the chickenpox vaccine.

NM: Chickenpox is usually a tame illness. The chickenpox vaccine was available for many years but authorities claimed it wasn't cost effective to promote it. Now authorities are prepared to license this vaccine because they finally came up with a winning pitch: think of all the money we'll save when parents won't have to stay at home to care for their sick children.[178] Financial arguments are poor rationales when considering our children's health.

Q. I remember growing up, and when one of us got chickenpox or measles, everybody got it, and that was the end of it. What is the purpose of creating a national environment in which we fear the natural responses of the immune system? Do we really believe that everyone would end up succumbing to disease?

NM: Somewhere along the line, confidence in the wisdom of the body was overrun by blind faith in medical dogma.

Q. What motivates the vaccine and medical industries?

NM: I believe the pharmaceutical companies and paid medical consultants are motivated by money, whereas average doctors are moved by fear — apprehension about their own extinction. Although some are aware of the problems with vaccines but are afraid to confront their superiors, many truly believe that if vaccination campaigns were halted, great epidemics would ravage society. Few trust the natural wonders of the body, even fewer believe in the existence of a superior being. This also explains why choices made by the "simpleminded masses" are intolerable.

Q. It always amazes me that we don't give God enough credit. He created the body and gave it the ability to heal on its own. Why do we believe that we need things forced into us?

NM: The body is a beautiful instrument of creation. With proper nutrition and lots of parental love, it can usually take care of itself.

Q. Are you aware of the Kefauver Amendments to the FDA Act that required drug manufacturers to prove the efficacy of their drugs by clinical trials before licensing? In 1972, the FDA interpreted these amendments as inapplicable to vaccine testing. In other words, vaccines are not required to be proven clinically effective before FDA approval.

NM: A lot of evidence suggests that the FDA is a hypocritical front for the medical establishment and pharmaceutical companies. Our country, for example, still relies on spurious studies that were done in Great Britain during the 1950s to determine the safety and efficacy of the dangerous pertussis vaccine.[179]

Q. That's because we have no control groups in our own population.

NM: The government doesn't require control groups. Such a requirement would imply that parents have a right to choose against the vaccines.

Q. How are vaccines made? What do they contain?

NM: I would be very surprised to find a doctor or health official willing to openly and honestly describe what goes into the production of vaccines that are being injected into our innocent and healthy children. The first ingredient is live viruses.

Q. Where do scientists get the live viruses? Do they produce them in a jar?

NM: Drug companies isolate the virus from infected matter. Some of the newer shots they're coming out with today are genetically engineered.

Q. They're injecting that right into the blood system?

NM: Yes, along with "stabilizing" agents: formaldehyde, which is a major component in embalming fluid; aluminum, a neurotoxin; and thimerosol, a mercury derivative.[180]

Q. Mercury, like in mercury poisoning?

NM: Yes, the same mercury that people are trying to remove from their teeth because of its toxic effects.

Q. Unbelievable!

NM: But first, this concoction needs to be incubated in living tissue. Scientists generally use animal organs. The polio vaccine, for example, is incubated in monkey kidneys. Monkeys are raised specifically for this purpose, to remove their kidneys. Chick embryos and human fetuses are also used.[181-183] This disgusting witch's brew is what gets injected into the child.

Q. That concoction sounds like voodoo.

NM: Or satanic ritualism, complete with child sacrifices.

Q. What do the animal activists think about using animals for vaccine production?

NM: Animal activists are generally opposed to any kind of animal experimentation. Vegetarians should also be outraged; very few are aware that when they dutifully take their children to a doctor for the shots, they're being injected with a product that was brewed in animal organs. Vaccines are not vegetarian.

Q. I was told the reason the children of the '60s were so crazy was that they had been vaccinated with material that had come from the monkey, that they had taken on simian characteristics. Have you heard that before?

NM: No, I haven't heard that theory before. But I do know that starting in the 1960s, learning disorders were being diagnosed in epidemic proportions, and national scholastic aptitude scores began a rapid decline.[184]

Q. I heard scientists may put the vaccines in vegetables.

NM: Yes, researchers are experimenting with vegetables and fruit. Soon, you may be able to eat a potato or banana to receive your vaccination.[185,186] It's shocking to consider, but biogenetic food engineering, where scientists cross-breed insect genes with our food supply, already exists.[187,188] And the FDA, while calling for more stringent labeling of harmless vitamins,[189] is refusing to let us know which foods are irradiated (treated with radiation) and which dairy products contain BGH, a bovine growth hormone injected into unfortunate cows and passed on to dairy consumers.[190]

Q. I heard that the World Health Organization laced a new tetanus vaccine with a birth control drug, then injected it into millions of women in Third World countries to control the population. Is this true?

NM: Human Life International (HLI), a Catholic human rights organization, recently published a disturbing report indicating that childbearing women in Mexico, the Philippines, and Nicaragua were injected with an anti-fertility vaccine without their consent or knowledge. They were simply told that they were receiving a new tetanus vaccine.[191]

Q. I live in an isolated area of Canada, and my children were not vaccinated. When they get sick, I'm not sure which childhood disease they may have, and I am reluctant to go to the doctor.

NM: I recommend Dr. Robert Mendelsohn's book, _How To Raise A Healthy Child...In Spite of Your Doctor_.[192] If you absolutely must take your child to a doctor, consider one of the many good holistic practitioners.

Q. How many doctors do you think support non-vaccination?

NM: Thousands of naturopathic, homeopathic, and chiropractic physicians are aware of the dangers associated with vaccines. They recommend alternative approaches to achieving health.

Q. Were your children vaccinated?

NM: No.

Q. What does your family doctor have to say about raising your children without vaccinations?

NM: My children have never been to a doctor. They were born at home with the support of a midwife. And because they don't receive vaccines, antibiotics, or other immune-depleting drugs, they're rarely sick.

Q. What is your family diet like?

NM: We eat organically grown food as much as possible, and we try to avoid animal products, sugar, and preservatives.

Q. Are you feeling any pressure while speaking out against mandated vaccines and for writing on this subject? Are you ever afraid for yourself or your family?

NM: My friends have warned me that the opposition can be ruthless. But people have been speaking out against vaccines since the concept was introduced. I merely advocate freedom of choice. It is immoral to mandate vaccines when one considers all the conflicting information that exists regarding their safety and efficacy.

Q. How do vaccinations and immunizations differ, or are they the same thing?

NM: I regard the term "immunizations" as a misnomer because vaccines have poor efficacy rates. Breastfed babies are immunized, whereas children who receive the shots are vaccinated.

Q. How do epidemics differ from outbreaks?

NM: An epidemic implies numerous instances of a disease; an outbreak, on the other hand, refers to a sudden increase in the number of cases. No matter how a disease is labeled in the media, try to ascertain how many instances of it are occurring in vaccinated versus unvaccinated people.

Q. Whatever happened to the bubonic plague, a very contagious and fatal disease?

NM: The plague killed many people in its time. There wasn't a vaccine to "prevent" it, yet it's essentially gone.

Q. I understand that the spread of the plague had to do with sewage running through the middle of towns. It had to do with poor sanitation.

NM: Several diseases declined on their own before the vaccines were introduced.[193] Increased nutritional and sanitary awareness is a likely explanation.[194-198]

Q. I once read that prisoners were promised their freedom if they agreed to bury victims of the plague. Well, they ate garlic paste for three days, performed the task, and none of them died.

NM: A powerful testament to the interrelationship between diet and health.

Q. I noticed that smallpox vaccinations are no longer required for overseas travel.

NM: Smallpox vaccinations were recently discontinued throughout the world. In fact, scientists are currently debating whether or not to destroy the last laboratory vials of the disease.[199]

Q. Are any vaccines required before traveling to other countries?

NM: No. Although some shots may be suggested, they are rarely "required" for travel abroad. Nor are vaccinations required upon returning to the United States. Nevertheless, Americans planning trips abroad are often led to believe the shots are required. Ironically, some people get so sick after receiving these "health-protecting" germs that they never make it out of the States.

Q. I had to have vaccinations before going to Argentina to serve a mission for my church. Needless to say, I was never able to fulfill my call. Shortly after receiving the shots I contracted an undiagnosed illness. I have been suffering for the past three years. I have been to every kind of doctor, to no avail. The conventional doctors simply tell me I am crazy.

NM: I'm sorry to hear of your unfortunate incident.

Q. What about the major diseases? Is it safe to travel abroad without vaccinations?

NM: When medical authorities believe there is a concern, they inform travelers of their recommendations. Then, people may use their discretion regarding the vaccines.

Q. What about vaccinations for our pets?

NM: New vaccines for animal diseases are developed and promoted on a regular basis. Recently, a very concerned animal lover told me that she thinks the new vaccines are damaging the immune systems of domesticated pets, especially purebred animals. Others have voiced their concerns that when a child's pet is vaccinated, the disease germ may be transferred to the child.[200] This possibility needs to be explored.

Q. My puppy is very sick. Our veterinarian says he has Parvo, which is a serious canine disease. But this same veterinarian recently vaccinated our puppy against Parvo. He said the vaccine doesn't always work. Now it's going to cost me hundreds of dollars to get my dog well again.

NM: Your vet said the vaccine doesn't always work. A more likely explanation is that the vaccine gave your puppy the disease. I recommend _Dr. Pitcairn's Complete Guide to Natural Health for Dogs and Cats._

Q. What alternatives are there to vaccines? Is there something that can be taken to ward off these diseases?

NM: I recommend consulting with a holistic health practitioner. I also endorse getting your newborn off to a great start in life with breastmilk, fresh air, a secure emotional environment, and lots of skin-to-skin contact. When the baby is weaned, offer only natural, organic foods. Avoid sugar and unnecessary additives, because research indicates they may break down the immune system.[201,202]

Q. Thank you for giving our children a voice, for educating parents, and for speaking out on this very important topic.

NM: You're welcome.

NOTES

1. Michael Alderson, *International Mortality Statistics: Facts on File* (Washington, DC, 1981), pp. 177-178.

2. *Physicians' GenRx,* (New York: Data Pharmaceutica, 1993), p. II-1691.

3. V. A. Jegede, et al., "Vaccine Technology," *Encyclopedia of Chemical Technology,* (New York: John Wiley and Sons, 1983), pp. 628-630.

4. Jamie Murphy, "The Making of a Vaccine," *What Every Parent Should Know About Childhood Immunization,* (Boston: Earth Healing Products, 1993), pp. 25-28.

5. *Report of the Committee on Infectious Diseases, 1986* (American Academy of Pediatrics), pp. 284-285.

6. Peter M. Strebel, et al, "Epidemiology of Polio in the U.S. One Decade after the Last Reported Case of Indigenous Wild Virus Associated Disease," *Clinical Infectious Diseases,* (Centers for Disease Control, February 1992), pp. 568-79.

7. Ibid.

8. Ibid.

9. Hearings before the Committee on Interstate and Foreign Commerce, House of Representatives, 87th Congress, 2nd Session on HR 10541, May 1962, pp. 94-112.

10. Christopher Kent, DC, PhD, "Drugs, Bugs, and Shots in the Dark," *Health Freedom News,* (January 1983), p. 26.

11. Richard Moskowitz, MD, "Immunizations: The Other Side," *Vaccinations: The Rest of The Story,* (Santa Fe, NM: Mothering, 1992), p. 86.

12. Robert Gallo, *Virus Hunting: AIDS, Cancer, & the Human Retrovirus,* (Harper Collins, 1991), pp. 28-29.

13. "Vaccine Safety Committee Proceedings [Transcripts]," *Institute of Health,* (Washington, DC: National Academy of Sciences, May 11, 1992), p. 13.

14. Tom Curtis, "The Origin of AIDS: A Startling New Theory Attempts to Answer the Question 'Was it an Act of God or an Act of Man,'" *Rolling Stone,* (March 19, 1992), pp. 54+.

15. Walter S. Kyle, "Simian retroviruses, poliovaccine, and origin of AIDS," *Lancet,* (March 7, 1992), pp. 600-601.

16. Eva Lee Snead, MD, *Some Call it AIDS: I Call it Murder,* (San Antonio, Texas: AUM Publications, 1992), p. 36.

17. William Campbell Douglass, MD, "WHO Murdered Africa," *Health Freedom News,* (September 1987), p. 42.

18. Eva Lee Snead, MD, "AIDS — Immunization Related Syndrome," *Health Freedom News,* (July 1987), p. 1

19. William Bennett, *The Atlantic Monthly,* (Harvard University Press: February, 1976).

20. "Division of Biologics Standards: The Boat That Never Rocked," *Science,* (March 17, 1972).

21. Arthur J. Snider, "Near Disaster with the Salk Vaccine," *Science Digest,* (1963).

22. B. L. Horvath, et al., "Excretion of SV-40 virus after oral administration of contaminated polio vaccine," *Acta Microbiologica Hungary,* 11, pp. 271-275.

23. N. P. Thompson, et al., "Is Measles Vaccination a Risk Factor for Inflammatory Bowel Disease?," *Lancet,* (April 29, 1995), pp. 1071-1074.

24. C. M. Benjamin, et al., "Joint and Limb Symptoms in Children After Immunisation With Measles, Mumps, and Rubella Vaccine," *British Medical Journal,* (April 25, 1992), p. 1075-1078.

25. Roland W. Sutter, et al., "Attributable Risk of DTP Injection in Provoking Paralytic Poliomyelitis During a Large Outbreak in Oman," *The Journal of Infectious Disease,* (March 1992), pp. 444-449.

26. L. Herroelen, et al., "Central Nervous System Demyelination After Immunization with Recombinant Hepatitis B Vaccine," *Lancet,* 338, (1991), pp. 1174-1175.

27. Michel Garenne, et al., "Child Mortality After High-Titre Measles Vaccines: Prospective Study in Senegal," *Lancet,* (October 12, 1991), pp. 903+.

28. Dr. A.D. Lieberman, "The Role of the Rubella Virus in the Chronic Fatigue Syndrome," *Clinical Ecology*, Vol. 7, No. 3, pp. 51-54.

29. Dr. Allen B. Allen, "Is RA27/3 a Cause of Chronic Fatigue?" *Medical Hypothesis*, 27 (1988), pp. 217-220.

30. Viera Scheibner, PhD, *Vaccination: 100 Years of Orthodox Research Shows That Vaccines Represent a Medical Assault on the Immune System*, (Australia, 1993).

31. Harris L. Coulter, *Vaccination, Social Violence, and Criminality: The Medical Assault on the American Brain*, (Berkeley, CA: North Atlantic Books, 1990).

32. M. Burnet and D. White, *The Natural History of Infectious Disease* (Cambridge, 1972), p. 16.

33. Benjamin P. Sandler, MD, *Diet Prevents Polio*, (The Lee Foundation for Nutritional Research, 1951).

34. See Note 1.

35. See Note 33.

36. See Note 32.

37. See Notes 14-22.

38. See Notes 12 and 13.

39. See Note 1, pp. 182-183.

40. See Note 11.

41. Daniel Q. Haney, "Wave of Infant Measles Stems From '60s Vaccinations," *Albuquerque Journal*, (November 23, 1992), p. B3.

42. Ibid.

43. *FDA Workshop to Review Warnings, Use Instructions, and Precautionary Information [on Vaccines]*, (Rockville, Maryland, Sept. 18, 1992), p. 37.

44. Groupe médical de Réflexion sur le vaccin ROR, "The Immunization Campaign Against Measles, Mumps, and Rubella, Coercion Leading to a Realm of Uncertainty: Medical Objections to a Continued MMR Immunization Campaign in Switzerland," *JAM, Vol 9, No. 1*, (1992), p. 7.

45. *National Health Federation Bulletin*, (November 1969).

46. See Note 44, pp. 5 and 6.

47. Harold E. Buttram, MD, "Foreword By...," *Vaccines: Are They Really Safe and Effective? A Parent's Guide To Childhood Shots*, (Santa Fe, New Mexico: New Atlantean Press, 1994), pp. 9-11.

48. Robert S. Mendelsohn, MD, *Immunizations: The Terrible Risks Your Children Face That Your Doctor Won't Reveal*, (Second Opinion Publishing, 1993), p. 88.

49. Dr. Beverley Allan, *Australian Nurses Journal*, (May 1978).

50. See Notes 28 and 29.

51. *Adverse Effects of Pertussis and Rubella Vaccines*, (Washington, DC: National Academy Press, 1991).

52. Sam Biser, "Chronic Fatigue Syndrome," *The Last Chance Health Report*, Volume 3, No. 7, (1993), pp. 1-6. Also see Notes 28 and 29.

53. Ibid.

54. See Note 6.

55. Edward Mortimer, "Immunization Against Infectious Disease," *Science*, Volume 200, (May 26, 1978), p. 905.

56. Richard Moskowitz, "Unvaccinated Children," *Mothering* (Winter 1987), p. 36.

57. *New England Journal of Medicine*, (July 7, 1994), pp. 16-19.

58. See Note 11.

59. *Whooping Cough, the DPT Vaccine and Reducing Vaccine Reactions* (Vienna, VA: National Vaccine Information Center, 1989). Also see Note 30, pp. 13-79.

60. Harris L. Coulter and Barbara Loe Fisher, *A Shot in the Dark: Why the P in DPT Vaccination May be Hazardous to Your Child's Health*, (Garden City Park, NY: Avery Publishing Group, 1991), pp. 208-210.

61. Carl Scully, M.P., *Immunisation: Is It Worth The Risk?*, (Fairfield, England: Scully, 1992), pp. 116.

62. Ibid.

63. See Note 30, p. 41.

64. Ibid. p. 33.

65. Fine and Chen, "Confounding in Studies of Adverse Reactions to Vaccines," *American Journal of Epidemiology*, 136, (1992), pp. 121-35.

66. Dr. Viera Scheibnerova, *Cot Death as Due to Exposure to Non-Specific Stress and General Adaption Syndrome: Its Mechanisms and Prevention*, (New South Wales, Australia: Association for Prevention of Cot Death, October 1990).

67. W. C. Torch, "Diphtheria-Pertussis-Tetanus (DPT) Immunization: A Potential Cause of the Sudden Infant Death Syndrome (SIDS)," (American Academy of Neurology,

34th Annual Meeting, Apr 25 - May 1, 1982), *Neurology* 32(4), pt. 2.

68. See Note 31, pp. xiii-xiv; chapters 1-5.

69. Richard Leviton, "A Shot in the Dark," *Yoga Journal,* (May/June, 1992), p. 128.

70. *Journal of the American Medical Association,* (August 24/31, 1994), pp. 592-593.

71. National Vaccine Injury Compensation Program, "Monthly Status Report," ($522 million spent as of February 3, 1995).

72. See Note 30, pp. 30 and 31.

73. See Note 61.

74. "Morbidity and Mortality Weekly Report Summary of Notifiable Diseases," *National Center for Health Statistics Mortality Reports,* (1992).

75. See Note 61.

76. See Note 30, pp. 13-79; also see Notes 59, 66, and 67.

77. See Note 11, p. 91.

78. See Note 67.

79. See Note 66.

80. *NVIC Mini News.* (Vienna, VA: National Vaccine Information Center, November 1990), p. 3.

81. Eleanor McBean, *The Poisoned Needle,* (Mokelumne Hill, CA: Health Research, 1957), pp. 12,13.

82. William White, *The Story of a Great Delusion,* (London: E.W. Allen, 1885), p. xi. Also see Note 81, pp. 5-85.

83. See Note 81, p. 64. Also see Note 82, p. xxxv.

84. "'Meningitis' Vaccine is Really Not...," *Pediatric Patter,* (Aug. 1986).

85. See Note 48, p. 5.

86. Sydney S. Gellis, MD, ed., *Pediatric Notes: The Weekly Pediatric Commentary,* Volume 11:2, (January 15, 1987).

87. Robert S. Mendelsohn, MD, "New Vaccine to Combat Day Care Infections," *The People's Doctor Newsletter,* (Volume 9, No. 11), p. 5. (Figures reported by Dr. Stephen L. Coeni of the Centers for Disease Control).

88. "Meningitis Risk Seen from Use of Vaccine," *St. Paul Pioneer Press Dispatch,* (April 21, 1987).

89. R. Weiss, "Meningitis Vaccine Stirs Controversy," *Science News,* Volume 132, (October 24, 1987), p. 260.

90. Robert S. Mendelsohn, MD, "The Drive to Immunize Adults is On," *Herald of Holistic Health Newsletter,* (September-October, 1985), p. 2.

91. *Boston Globe,* (June 11, 1991), p. 1F; *Pharmaceutical Rep.,* (Mar. 1992); *NVIC News,* (National Vaccine Information Center, Vienna, VA., April 1992), p. 12.

92. Ibid.

93. Richard Moskowitz, MD, "Vaccination: A Sacrament of Modern Medicine." Presented in a speech at the Annual Conference of the Society of Homeopaths, (Manchester, England, September 1991), p. 6.

94. See Note 48, p. 75.

95. Ibid.

96. "Bad Flu Season Forecast; Elderly Urged to Get Shots Now," *The New Mexican,* (October 1, 1993), p. B6.

97. Ibid.

98. "Vaccine Safety Committee Proceedings [Transcripts]," *Institutes of Health,* (Washington, DC: National Academy of Sciences, May 11, 1992), pp. 14-19.

99. See Note 96.

100. See Note 48, p. 4.

101. See Notes 9 and 10.

102. See Note 90.

103. See Notes 14-22.

104. H. H. Merritt, *Textbook of Neurology,* Sixth Edition, (Philadelphia, PA: Lea and Febiger, 1979), p. 104.

105. Josephine B. Neal, *Encephalitis: A Clinical Study,* (New York: Grune and Stratton, 1942), pp. 378-379.

106. Anna Lisa Annell, "Pertussis in Infancy — A Cause of Behavioral Disorders in Children," *Acta Societatis Medicorum Upsaliensis,* XVIII, Supplement 1, (1953), pp. 17, 33.

107. A. B. Baker, "The Central Nervous System in Infectious Diseases of Childhood," *Postgraduate Medicine,* 5, (1949), p. 11.

108. Lurie, et al, "Late Results Noted in Children Presenting Post-Encephalitic Behavior," *American Journal of Psychiatry,* 104, (1947), p. 178.

109. Frank R. Ford, *Diseases of the Nervous System in Infancy, Childhood, and Adolescence,* (Springfield: C. C. Thomas, 1937), p. 349.

110. *Physicians' Desk Reference*, (Montvale, New Jersey: Medical Economics Data Production, 1995). Also see Note 2.

111. See Note 44, pp. 5 and 6. Also see Note 47.

112. Harold E. Buttram, MD and John Chriss Hoffman, *Vaccinations and Immune Malfunction*, (Quakertown, PA: The Randolph Society, 1985).

113. See Note 44, pp. 5 and 6. Also see Note 47.

114. See Note 30, p. 49.

115. See Note 51.

116. See Notes 28, 29, and 52.

117. Michel Garenne, et al., "Child Mortality After High-titre Measles Vaccines: Prospective Study in Senegal," *The Lancet*, Volume 338, (October 12, 1991), pp. 903-907.

118. Ibid., p. 906.

119. Jane M. Healy, PhD, *Endangered Minds: Why Our Children Don't Think*, (New York: Simon & Schuster, Inc., 1990), pp. 13-35.

120. See Note 31.

121. Ibid.

122. Leo Kanner, "Autistic Disturbances of Affective Content," *The Nervous Child II*, (1942-1943), p. 250.

123. American Psychiatric Association, *Diagnostic and Statistical Manual of Mental Disorders*, Third Edition, Revised, (Washington, DC, 1987), pp. 36-37.

124. S. Wakabayashi, "The Present Status of an Early Infantile Autism First Reported in Japan 30 Years Ago," *Nagoya Medical Journal*, 46, (1984), pp. 35+.

125. See Note 31, p. 50.

126. V. S. Cowart, "Attention-Deficit Hyperactivity Disorder: Physicians Helping Parents Pay More Heed," *Journal of American Medical Association*, 259:18, (May 13, 1988), p. 2647.

127. D. M. Ross and S. A. Ross, *Hyperactivity: Research, Theory, and Action*, (New York: John Wiley, 1982).

128. Kathleen Long and D.V. Queen, "Detection and Treatment of Emotionally Disturbed Children in Public Schools: Problems and Theoretical Perspectives," *Journal of Clinical Psychology*, 40:1, (January 1984), p. 378.

129. See Note 31, p. 50. Also see Notes 123 and 124.

130. See Notes 14 and 15.

131. See Note 17.

132. Ibid.

133. Department of Defense Appropriations for 1970: Hearings before a Subcommittee of the Committee on Appropriations, House of Representatives, Ninety-First Congress, First Session, (June 9, 1969), p. 129.

134. *London Times*, (May 11, 1987), p. 1.

135. "AIDS Vaccine Study in Peril," *Chicago Tribune*, (May 29, 1994), p. 1.

136. *Vaccine Exemptions: A State-by-State Summary of Legal Exemptions to 'Mandatory' Vaccine Laws*, (Santa Fe, New Mexico: New Atlantean Press, 1995).

137. HR 940 (February 17, 1993); Senate Bills 732 and 733 (April 1, 1993).

138. In a statement made by President Clinton at a *Reading of Immunization Proclamation* on April 11, 1993. In a White House Press Release, April 12, 1993.

139. National Vaccine Injury Compensation Program, "Monthly Status Report," (Through February 3, 1995).

140. H.R. 78, 103rd Congress, 1st Session: A Bill, (January 5, 1993).

141. H.R. 1840 103rd Congress, 1st Session: A Bill, (April 22, 1993).

142. See Note 140.

143. "Concerned Parents Unfairly Shut Out of Congressional Hearings on Vaccines," *Dayton Daily News*, (May 28, 1993), p. 15A.

144. In a September 16, 1990 letter written by Barbara Loe Fisher, to Donald A. Henderson, chairman of the National Vaccine Advisory Committee, p. 3.

145. See Note 139.

146. Vaccine Adverse Event Reporting System (VAERS), Rockville, Maryland.

147. "Why Am I So Sick?," *20-20 Newscast*, (January 26, 1990). Also see Note 141.

148. "What You Need to Know," (Atlanta, GA: CDC/U.S. Department of Health and Human Services).

149. "Congress to Investigate 10,000 Percent Increase in DPT Prices," (DPT News).

150. Ibid.

151. See Note 136.

152. See Note 141.

153. *Morbidity and Mortality Weekly Report*, (U.S. Govt., 39: 1990), pp. 353-363.

154. *Journal of the American Medical Association*, (June 26, 1991).

155. "Should You Vaccinate Against Measles?," *Natural Childcare*, (January/February 1992), p. 30.

156. *New England Journal of Medicine*, (July 7, 1994), pp. 16-21.

157. Michael W. Miller, "Efficacy of Whooping Cough Vaccines Is Questioned by Latest Research Data," *Wall Street Journal*, (July 7, 1994).

158. See Note 31. Also see Note 60, pp. 22-93.

159. See Note 59.

160. Compiled from multiple sources.

161. Senator John D. Rockefeller IV, Chair, "Is Military Research Hazardous to Veterans' Health? Lessons from the Cold War, the Persian Gulf, and Today: Opening Statement," *United States Senate, Committee on Veterans' Affairs* (May 6, 1994).

162. See Note 140, p. 2.

163. Robert Mendelsohn MD, *How To Raise A Healthy Child...In Spite of Your Doctor* (Chicago: Contemporary Books, 1984), pp. 210, 228.

164. *New England Journal of Medicine*, (July 7, 1994), pp. 16-21.

165. Michael W. Miller, "Efficacy of Whooping Cough Vaccines Is Questioned by Latest Research Data," *Wall Street Journal*, (July 7, 1994).

166. Halperin, et al. "Persistence of Pertussis in an Immunized Population: Results of the Nova Scotia Enhanced Pertussis Surveillance Program," *Journal of Pediatrics* (Nov. 1989), pp. 686-693.

167. *Vaccine Bulletin* (February 1987), p. 11.

168. *20th Immunization Conference Proceedings, Dallas, Texas, May 6-9, 1985*, (U.S. Department of Health and Human Services, October 1985), pp. 83-84.

169. Barkin and Pichichero, "Diphtheria-Pertussis-Tetanus Vaccine: Reactogenicity of Commercial Products," *Pediatrics* (Feb. 1979), pp. 256-260.

170. *Medical Tribune* (January 10, 1979), p. 1.

171. See Note 59, p. 3.

172. See Note 161.

173. Diana Zuckerman, PhD, and Patricia Olson, D.V.M., Ph.D., "Is Military Research Hazardous to Veterans' Health? Lessons from the Persian Gulf: Preliminary Staff Findings," *United States Senate, Committee on Veterans' Affairs*, (May 6, 1994).

174. See Note 147.

175. R. Weiss, "Breastmilk May Stimulate Immunity," *Science News*, (March 26, 1988), p. 196.

176. Lindsey Grossman, "Breastfeeding Healthier Babies," *USA Today*, (August 1988), p. 4.

177. Allan Cunningham, MD, "Breastfeeding and Health," *The Compleat Mother*, (Summer 1987), p. 36.

178. "Chickenpox Conundrum," *Time*, (July 19, 1993), p. 53.

179. See Note 60.

180. *Physicians' Desk Reference*, (Montvale, NJ: Medical Economics Data Production, 1995). Also see *Physicians' GenRx*, (New York: Data Pharmaceutica, 1993).

181. Ibid.

182. J. M. Hoskins and S. A. Plotkin, "Behaviour of Rubella Virus in Human Diploid Cell Strains," *Wistar Institute of Anatomy and Biology*, (Phila., PA: Jan. 16, 1969), pp. 284-295.

183. S. A. Plotkin, "Development of RA 27/3 Attenuated Rubella Virus Grown in WI-38 Cells," *International Symposium on Rubella Vaccines, London 1968; Symp. Series Immunobiological Standards*, Vol. 11, (Karger, Basel/New York, 1969), pp. 249-260.

184. See Note 119.

185. Carl Tant, *Awesome Green*, (Angleton, TX: Biotech Pub., 1994), pp. 108-115.

186. "Health Report," *Time*, (April 24, 1995), p. 17.

187. Sheldon Krimsky, "Tomatoes May Be Dangerous to Your Health," *The New York Times*, (June 1, 1992).

188. Deborah Houy, "Organica — Is Your Food Safe?" *Buzzworm: The Environmental Journal*, (September/October 1992).

189. John Morgenthaler, ed., *Stop the FDA*, (Menlo Park, CA: Health Freedom Publications, 1992).

190. See Note 187.

191. *HLI Reports* (June 1995); as reported in *The Vaccine Reaction*, (Vienna, VA: NVIC, July 1995), pp. 1-2.

192. See Note 163.

193. See Note 1.

194. "Virus Becomes Lethal With Poor Nutrition," *The New Mexican*, (May 1, 1995), p. A-2.

195. Orville Levander, *Nature Medicine*, (May 1, 1995).
196. See Note 33.
197. E. Douglas Hume, *Bechamp or Pasteur? A Lost Chapter in the History of Biology*, (London: C. W. Daniel & Company, 1923), pp. 127-128.
198. Michael Sheehan, "Was Pasteur Wrong?," *Natural Health*, (Jan/Feb 1992), pp. 41-44.
199. "Whispers of Fear Surround Last Vials of Smallpox," *Santa Fe, New Mexican*, (June 20, 1993), p. A1.
200. As reported by concerned parents and naturopathic veterinarians.
201. See Note 48, p. 96.
202. William Manahan, MD, *Eat For Health*, (Tiburon, CA: H.J. Kramer, Inc., 1988), pp. 60-76.

INDEX

New Atlantean Books

Additional copies of **Immunizations: The People Speak! —Questions, Comments, and Concerns About Vaccinations,** may be purchased directly from *New Atlantean Press*. Trade paperback, 80 pages, $8.95.

Other books available from New Atlantean Press:

Vaccines: Are They Really Safe and Effective? A Parent's Guide to Childhood Shots by Neil Z. Miller. Forewords by George R. Schwartz, M.D. and Harold E. Buttram, M.D. Can mandatory vaccines trigger developmental disorders and autoimmune diseases? Are they responsible for an unprecedented rise in criminal activity and violent crime? Did AIDS originate from diseased monkey organs used to incubate polio vaccines? Are new viruses tested on suspecting vaccine recipients? How safe is *your* child from the near and long-term effects of these "miracle" shots? This incredible vaccine handbook (50,000 copies sold!) systematically evaluates the safety, efficacy, and long-term effects of "mandatory" vaccines. It contains 12 diagrams and more than 300 references so that all of the data may be confirmed. Are vaccines *really* safe and effective? You be the judge. Trade paperback, 80 pages, 6th edition, 1-881217-10-8, $8.95.

Immunization Theory vs. Reality: Exposé on Vaccinations by Neil Z. Miller. Forewords by Dr. Lendon Smith, et al. This profound parenting and health resource contains the most compelling up-to-date information on vaccines (© 1996). It reads like a gut-wrenching investigational novel, gives voice to parents of vaccine-damaged children, lists exact ingredients in each vaccine, unravels the suppressed history of vaccines, and clarifies immune system development. This remarkable book also looks at natural health defenses, reveals the medical ploys used to hoodwink the public, and uncovers the truth behind the Gulf War Syndrome. Recent studies, as well as **solutions** to the vaccine dilemma, are provided. Includes complete documentation and a cross-referenced index. Do vaccine benefits *really* outweigh the risks? Discover the truth in this astonishing exposé. Trade paperback, 160 pages, 1-881217-12-4, © 1996, $12.95.

STATE VACCINE LAWS: Copies of the vaccine laws of YOUR state are now available. Don't allow yourself to be intimidated by overzealous authorities. Arm yourself with the **exact laws** of your state. 1-5p., $4.00.

Vaccine Exemptions: How to Legally Avoid Immunizations in All 50 States. Saddle-stitched booklet, 16 pages, regularly updated, $10.00.

ORDERING INFORMATION

These books may be purchased by sending the total amount, including 7% shipping ($3.50 minimum), to: **New Atlantean Press**, PO Box 9638-925, Santa Fe, NM 87504. Or call 505-983-1856 to order by credit card. A FREE catalog is included with every order.

P URCHASING INFORMATION

Additional copies of **Immunizations: The People Speak! —Questions, Comments, and Concerns About Vaccinations** (ISBN: 1-881217-16-7) may be purchased directly from *New Atlantean Press*. Send $8.95 (in U.S. funds), plus $3.50 shipping, to:

New Atlantean Press
PO Box 9638-925
Santa Fe, NM 87504

Vaccines: Are They Really Safe and Effective? A Parent's Guide to Childhood Shots (ISBN: 1-881217-10-8, 80p., 8.95), and **Immunization Theory vs. Reality: Exposé on Vaccinations** (ISBN: 1-881217-12-4, 160p., © 1996, 12.95), both by Neil Z. Miller, may also be purchased from *New Atlantean Press*.

These three books are also available at many fine bookstores.

Bookstores and Retail Buyers: Order from Baker & Taylor, Bookpeople, Ingram, New Leaf, Nutri-Books, or from New Atlantean Press. Libraries may order from your favorite library wholesaler.

Chiropractors, Homeopaths, Midwives, Naturopaths, Pediatricians, Vaccine Organizations, and other Non-Storefront Buyers: Take a 40% discount with the purchase of 5 or more copies (multiply the total cost of purchases x .60). Please add 7% ($3.50 minimum) for shipping.

Shipping: Books are usually shipped within 24 hours. Please allow one to three weeks for your order to arrive, or include $5.50 (for up to 2 books) for priority air mail shipping. Checks must be drawn on a U.S. bank, or send a Postal Money Order in U.S. funds. **Sales Tax:** Please add 6% for books shipped to New Mexico addresses.

FREE CATALOG: *New Atlantean Press* offers the world's largest selection of vaccine information, including up-to-date vaccination laws, vaccine books, and other hard to find vaccine resources imported from around the world. We also offer nearly 200 books and videos on cutting-edge alternative health solutions, natural immunity, progressive parenting, natural childcare, AIDS, cancer, and more. Send for a FREE CATALOG: New Atlantean Press, PO Box 9638-925, Santa Fe, NM 87504.

About the Author

Neil Miller is a research journalist and natural health advocate.